LIVE TO BE 180

LIVE TO BE

180

BY

JUSTINE C. GLASS

TAPLINGER PUBLISHING CO., INC.

NEW YORK

CONTENTS

v

LIVE TO BE 180

CHAPTER

1

YOU CAN LIVE TO BE 180

WHAT would you say is the normal span of human life?
Seventy or eighty years?

According to the computations of biologists, the life
span of any species is from seven to fourteen times the
period an individual of the species takes to reach maturity.
We mature between 20 and 25 years of age; our expectation of life could be 280, on that reckoning.

Some gerontologists ("old age" specialists) put it much
higher. Dr. Christopherson of London Hospital says: "A
man might live 300, 400, or even 1000 years, if the life-sustaining elements were present."

So a life span of 180 years is a very reasonable target.

First of all, let us establish that there is nothing freakish
in the idea of this length of life. It is only because it is

1

new to us that we are likely to think so. Scientists tell us that there is nothing in the nature of protoplasm which demands a wearing out. And humans, of course, are protoplasm.

Take a look at some of our relatives, who have been going—it's a fair assumption—almost since the beginning of time. There is the protoplasm called *Paramecium Aurelia,* or "immortal protoplasm." In 1911, L. L. Woodruff and R. Erdman began experiments with it. By 1928, 8000 generations had been registered, but it was still as good as new. It showed no sign of decay, senile or otherwise.

In the plant world, there is apparent "immortality" also. One of the cacti goes on living, it seems, forever. So do the giant sequoia trees of California. There are orange trees in the orangerie of the palace of Versailles said to have been planted by Eleanor of Castile. In Mexico there is a cypress which was a contemporary of Cortez. Baobabs, found chiefly in Africa, can live for 6000 years.

Some fish are Methuselahs. Carp and pike can live 300 years, if not indefinitely. A few hundred years is nothing to a crocodile—in Africa, crocodiles have been found which are believed to be about 1700 years old. Wild boars can live to about the 300-year mark; donkeys, swans and parrots are often centenarians. Tortoises sometimes survive for several centuries.

And even we, the human race, can put in a few records. Methuselah nearly reached Dr. Christopherson's suggested limit of 1000 years; according to the Old Testament, he was 969 when he died. Joseph lived to be 110, Sarah to 197, Abraham to 275. Moses, who began all this three-score-years-and-ten life-span business, lived to be 127 him-

self. And at that age, so the Bible says, "his eye was not
dim nor his natural force abated."

The ancient Greek race, the Pelasgians, would have considered that to die at 70 was to die in the cradle, almost.
Plato, Xenophon, and Pythagorus are among the writers
who tell us that Pelasgian life expectancy was at least 200
years. Like Moses, to the last their "natural force was not
abated." And their hair did not turn gray.

Galen, the great physician, lived 140 years. Socrates died
at 106 (and, but for that cup of hemlock, might have made
his second century), Sophocles at 130. Pliny tells us of a
musician who, at the age of 150, looked no more than 50.

Then there was the midwife who attended Henrietta
Maria, wife of Charles I; she lived to be 103. In 1500 a
man called Jenkins was born in Yorkshire. He died at the
age of 170. Thomas Parr's birthplace was London, the date
1588. He died 207 years later, also in London. There is a
record of a marriage which just missed a triple diamond
celebration. It lasted 147 years. The husband died at 173,
the wife at 184. At 150 years of age, these people are said
to have looked as if they were about 50.

Roger Bacon, who studied longevity, believed that a
man's span should be, normally, 1000 years.

In this century there are runners-up for this goal already. There are quite a few candidates in Russia, all well
on the far side of the first hundred years. In the Persian
village of Kelusah lives Sayed Ali, who is 195 years old.
He was married, he says, in 1790. His eldest son died
young—at 120—but Ali still has four children living. Two
sons are 105 and 90 respectively. He has a daughter of
110. The baby of the family, Gulbeenz, is 80. Sayed Ali is

fully active. He does not wear, and does not need to wear, spectacles.

Lyubov Pujak, a Russian, claims to be 150 years old and to have watched Napoleon's attack on Moscow. He has two younger brothers, aged 121 and 118, and a sister of only 112. In the Talysh mountains of Central Asia, Mahmoud Eivazov lives and works on a collective farm. Two years ago he was given the Red Banner of Labor on reaching his 148th birthday. He has 118 grandchildren, great-grand-children, and great-great-grandchildren.

A shooting contest, organized last year by the young people of the Caucasian village of Tsugari, was won by Mito Khubulov, who is 141 years of age.

Several American Civil War veterans survived both the fighting and the century mark, and some former slaves were alive and sprightly at between 115 and 120.

Not yet in the same class, but coming up well, is a Mrs. de Vere of Canterbury, Britain, who on her 103rd birth-day last year cooked lunch for her children, grandchildren, and great-grandchildren—and got up extra early to make sure that everything ran according to plan. Among the people following the longevity plan outlined in this book is a woman of 75. She teaches a strenuous form of dancing; she is as supple as a girl in her twenties—and looks as if she were in her forties. Her flesh is firm; she has no wrinkles. Her hair is dark; her teeth are beautiful—and her own.

Slim, trim, and active is a woman I know of, whose hair is light brown and whose complexion is attractive at 85. Last year she had three proposals of marriage. But she is still single; she said she would "wait a bit before taking the plunge."

A doctor was mistaken for his own son by a woman he had treated forty years before.

Miss Marion Jones wrote her autobiography, *The Jottings of Jemima,* two years ago when she was 100. Not too long afterward, her neighbors complained of the noise in her flat because of the number of visitors. So Miss Jones moved to a house outside Edinburgh, Scotland, where she could entertain undisturbed and undisturbing.

There is nothing bizarre, I repeat, in living out one's full life span. The people who do it are neither freaks nor helpless hulks. It is only because we do not yet meet men and women every day who are over 100 that we find anything odd about living to such an age. We shall get used to it. If you were a crocodile, you would not think twice about the fact that your father was over 1000. Nor would you expect him to be a senile invalid.

It is only because we have been conditioned to a lifetime of three score years and ten that to live longer, and to live longer without growing old, seems so fantastic. It is because the tempo of our minds is set to a shorter rhythm that we feel a life span of 180 years would be endless. But in any case, why worry now about whether time will drag when you're in your hundreds? You can start complaining then if you find the days too long—but by then you will never find time to do all you want to do.

It is a fact that, as we grow older, time passes more quickly. Do you remember how, when you were a child, a month seemed to last about as long as a year lasts now? And that a school term stretched to eternity?

Both physiologically and psychologically, much more happens to us when we are young than when we get older.

So a year to a child is really much longer than it is to an adult. It has been estimated that sidereal time flows four times slower for a child of 10 than for a man of 50. "Young and old," says Pierre Lecomte du Noüy, "united in the same space, live in separate universes, where the value of time is radically different."

Who hasn't said, "If only I had time to do so and so . . ."? Most of us have to leave so much undone. By the time we have managed to get enough knowledge and experience and poise to enjoy life, it is almost over.

If the great philosophers and scientists and leaders of world progress had had a little more time, the human race might be much better off in many ways than it now is. Guglielmo Marconi, the inventor of wireless telegraphy, said: "Life is too short." But, he added, "I think that hygiene and biochemistry will teach mankind to prolong its years far beyond the three score and ten."

Well, we *are* learning. Hygiene has disposed of some threats to longevity. Biochemistry (the science of life) is showing what the natural resources of foodstuffs can do toward increasing the length of youth and life.

The great American nutritionist, Professor Henry C. Sherman, has shown that the life span of animals can be increased enormously by correct diet—the supply of the foods which contain elements necessary to the processes of the body. Sherman says that never before have we known so much about our bodies' needs, so that never before have we been in a better position to supply them, a point which I shall refer to again. By correct diet we too can lay the foundations of a longer life span for ourselves.

Many people have the mistaken idea that we cannot live long or healthily unless we "get back to Nature." But how far back? Are we to swing from the trees by a substitute for our now nonexistent tails? Or find ourselves a fur wrap and a cave? Or retire to a log cabin without benefit of electricity or plumbing?

Surely the conditions of the age in which we happen to live are "natural" for us, and it is common sense to make use of their benefits when we can. That does not mean to say we need accept the mistakes as well—among them the processed foods and the impure air. We can get something done to put these right—if we try hard enough and long enough.

And meanwhile, among the benefits of our age, we have opportunities of improving physical health in ways not available to our ancestors. Sherman has exploded the idea that primitive man necessarily lived healthily, that his diet was "right." Primitive man could not pick and choose what he would have for dinner. He ate what he could get on the spot—and that was that. Perhaps it was right; in terms of nutritional needs, perhaps it wasn't. That often it wasn't is demonstrated by the condition of prehistoric skeletons. "Post-mortems" on them show many forms of imperfection, including dental cavities.

Our early ancestors went short of minerals and vitamins. Now we need not go short of them. We can build up health in ways not possible in those days. In a few years, scientists say, dental caries should occur no more often than rickets occurs today.

We can help our bodies to keep going for the full biologic span by providing right conditions, says Dr. Edward Börtz, former president of the American Medical Association. He believes that our life span should be a minimum of 150 years. The conditions essential to achieving it he lists as exercise, a straight spine, good diet, plenty of meat, eggs, and milk; vitamins and minerals, and two to three quarts of liquid daily—enough sleep and rest, and occupation for mind and hands.

But there is another factor, the vital factor. It is YOU— your attitude to life, your will to live. Dr. Börtz stresses this point. "It largely depends on each individual how long he or she lives," he says.

This onward-thrusting force has been operating since it sent protoplasm in search of better living quarters and urged fish to quit the water and grow wings. It is in all of us, and it can help us to claim the birthright of our normal span of life, *if we awaken it.*

Although we all have it, we don't all use our will to live. This accounts for the fact that some people go on when others stop, that some people are living although their doctors say they should be dead.

> One ship sails east and another west
>   With the self-same winds that blow;
> 'Tis the set of the sail and not the gale
>   Which determines the way they go.

We have to set our sails toward the 180 mark if we want to reach it. We have to believe we can achieve it, and make every effort to that end. As Dr. Börtz says: People must help themselves as well as take advantage of scientific discoveries.

Living to be 180 is a matter of making full use of all these discoveries and of all our potentialities, mental and physical. It can reveal us to ourselves, because so few of us have any idea of the scope of our full capabilities and energies. We can all surprise ourselves by what we can do when we really try.

The body is a superb, self-renewing organism. Give it the tools and it will do its job. But you can't make bricks without straw—and that is what most people seem to expect their bodies to do.

The mind is a dynamo, capable of generating a power, the limits of which no one so far can even guess.

Every one of us is well equipped to set out on the adventure of achieving longevity. Our ancestors, who won their battle for survival, saw to that.

The next step is up to you.

SUMMARY

MOSES' PRESCRIPTION of 70 as the cut-off point for the human life span has been followed by centuries of uncritical acceptance. Yet, in the words of a song from *Porgy and Bess,* "It ain't necessarily so!" Moses himself disproved it by departing, according to the Old Testament, vigorous at 127.

In the world of nature

- the *Paramecium Aurelia* has been living almost since the beginning of time
- the baobab can live 6000 years
- today's sequoia trees include many that are centuries old
- crocodiles believed to be 1700 years old have been found

- wild boars, carp, and pike can live at least 300 years
- even the jackass joins the century club

Among humans

- the Bible says that Methuselah lived 969 years, Abraham 275, and his wife Sarah reached 197
- the Pelasgians of ancient Greece had a life expectancy of 200
- Thomas Parr, a Londoner, lived to be 207
- an Iranian, Sayed Ali, is presently living his way from the age of 195 to 200
- a considerable number of people today are over 100 and going strong

In view of all this, and the fact that knowledgeable physicians could live from 300 to 1000 years, even 180 is a modest goal!

CHAPTER

2

CONQUEST OF DECAY

THE fight is on.

All over the world scientists and medical men have joined against the forces of decay and death. In laboratories, in clinics, at world conferences, they are discovering, discussing, experimenting with ways and means of defeating senility and extending the human life span.

"Freedom from senility is possible," says Dr. Martin Gumpert, a leading American gerontologist. "Old age is a disease, and it is curable," Professor H. C. Sherman, the eminent nutritionist, tells us. Metalnikov, the famous Russian biologist, has said: "It is possible to delay old age and death, and science must take a very serious interest in this problem."

New scientific discoveries constantly reaffirm these statements. Medical opinion confirms them. Doctors say: "With

11

our aggregate of medical knowledge, no child need suffer from rickets, and no elderly person need suffer from senility." "Census statistics show clearly that prolongation of productive life is not a Utopian dream." Finally, "There is no truth either to the formula that we must die at 70, or to the belief that we must necessarily be tortured in old age by the humiliation of senility."

That is certainly clear enough, isn't it?

Take particular note of the first part of the last-quoted medical opinion. It is another nail in the coffin of the three-score-years-and-ten myth—and it is about time that this was decently buried. For centuries we have been hypnotized by the idea that seventy years of life is our allotted span. For this, as I said earlier, Moses was to blame to a great extent. His recorded pronouncement was probably the greatest single source of discouragement to would-be "longer-lifers."

The average person has long considered that living beyond the age of seventy was a fluke, a freakish notion— flying in the face of Providence. Yet Moses himself is said to have lived to be 127. And in the book of Genesis we find these words: "The Lord said . . . 'man also is flesh, yet his days shall be 120 years.' "

It is odd that we should prefer to believe Moses rather than the Creator in this matter. After all, He should know. Yet most of us plan our lives to fit in with the seventy-year span. It is the basis of insurance companies' policies. Pension plans and retirement ages are geared to it. You and I and our parents were brought up and educated to this pattern, as are children today. It is firmly established in the human mind.

An idea which is accepted hook, line, and sinker by the

mind becomes a force to be reckoned with. It sinks into the subconscious. It can influence behavior; it can affect the tissues of the body. Doctors acknowledge this when they admit the important part a patient's attitude and convictions play in recovery from illness or in keeping disease at bay.

So, a belief in the seventy-year allotted span must be cleared thoroughly away before we can make real progress toward our 180th birthdays. Doubt can sabotage all our efforts. It can lose any battle for us by undermining our forces from within.

If you want to get results, from this moment onward refuse to give houseroom in your mind to negative thoughts for one single moment. The thoughts that age is creeping up on you, that disease is waiting around the corner, that you are weakening or deteriorating in any way must not be allowed to register in the subconscious. They are dangerous, they act as poisons in the mind, they materialize as real obstacles in the path of achievement. Begin to think and act and plan NOW for a long life, for long health and long youth. These concepts will crowd out failure thoughts. The mind cannot hold two ideas simultaneously.

Science assures us that there is no reason why we should not realize our full life potential. But we, ourselves, must also be convinced that it can be done. This is the basis on which, to a great extent, success depends.

The mind needs time to accustom itself to fresh ideas. Give your new attitude a chance to jell. And constantly remind yourself that you are laying the foundations of long health and youth and life, and that what you are doing must produce the results you want.

Sooner or later the prospect of living to 180 will be

generally accepted, and it will seem no more remarkable than the thought of living to 80 is at the moment. Longevity is a trend. It is developing with another trend: the trend of nations to age—the proportion of old to young people in most nations is increasing rapidly.

In Britain, by the end of 1961, according to estimates, the number of people over 65 will be 5,300,000. In the United States, there are today, according to the latest published figures, more than 15,300,000 people who are over 65. If those twenty million plus are to be "passengers" —if they are less and less able to pull their weight in the life of the nation—productive workers will have to carry a crippling burden. And there will be other problems, also. If people get old at 65 and become more and more infirm in their seventies and eighties, and if the numbers in these age groups increase, the number of younger people needed to look after them must increase also.

That will mean a two-way whittling down of manpower. The proportion of active workers in the population will be smaller—and a substantial number of them will not be available for essential industries. They will be needed to look after the old people.

In any language and any country, this is a problem. If the productive life of men and women could be prolonged, that would be an answer. That is one reason why the fight against decay has become a global warfare, and why the possibilities of living long without growing old are being probed all over the world.

A congress of medical men was held in London recently to discuss the subject. In Basle, about a year ago, a hundred doctors recorded their opinion that "to show signs of aging at 80 is premature," and that "we should live to at least 140 years of age, or more."

America has a Life Prolongation Research Institute, headed by Dr. Johan Björksten. He is a biochemist and a gerontologist; his researches are subsidized by the U.S. Air Force Scientific Research Department to the amount of some $8500 a year. The reason for this is that the cost of training a pilot is so high and his operational life so short that it is not an economic proposition. The USAF considers it well worth while to subsidize research which might make the extension of a man's flying years possible.

Dr. Björksten, a 46-year-old Swedish scientist, believes that we grow old because, as we go through life, molecules of protein of which all cells are made—and which they must have for repair and maintenance and rebuilding—become interlocked. In that condition they cannot be used by the system. They form useless "dumps" which clog the cells. This cluttering of the system with ineffective protein, says Dr. Björksten, results in aging and in death.

Dr. Björksten is trying to discover a substance which is capable of breaking up this cross-linkage of molecules. Then the body's machinery would be in running order once more. And when (Dr. Björksten says *when,* not *if*) it is discovered, people will stop growing old and begin growing younger. "It may prove easier to reverse the aging process than to halt it," he says.

Nutritionists have always been in the forefront of the fight against decay. A world-famous pioneer of the "science of eating," Professor Henry C. Sherman, who has already been quoted, has proved by experiments with animals that certain vitamins and minerals, when added to a normal diet, can extend the length of life and also the prime of life. Dr. Tom Spies, another great name in nutrition, has been working for more than twenty years along these lines. He has treated prematurely aged men and women, and invalids who have been given up by doctors as hopeless cases. The treatment used has been "food therapy"—diets high in protein, natural vitamins, and minerals, supplemented by synthetic vitamins. Dr. Spies says that the renewed health and vitality of these people show that "premature aging can be reversed and the period of the prime prolonged."

Dr. T. S. Gardner, another internationally known nutrition expert, has proved the importance of food to longevity. He found that the life span of animals could be increased by 46.4 per cent by the addition of pyridoxin (Vitamin B_6), yeast nucleic acid, and pantothexic acid (another B vitamin) to their diet.

The fight against decay must include campaigns against "killer" diseases. Dr. F. Steigman of Chicago, Dr. Charles Glen King, Director of the Nutrition Foundation of New York City, and Charles West of Toronto, one of the discoverers of insulin, are among the pioneers of research into the prevention of abnormal accumulations of fatty substances in the liver and elsewhere. These fatty deposits are thought to be directly related to the incidence of the chief killers of our time: heart attacks, strokes, and kidney disease. Thirty-five per cent of the population of England over the age of 10 died from vascular diseases in 1946, and the number is still rising. In another chapter, we shall go into this matter in greater detail.

The chief treatment used in such cases was a high-protein diet, with massive vitamin dosage, particularly of one of the B group, choline. This vitamin is usually present in most diets in borderline amounts only. It is one of the factors that controls fat movement in the body, the lipotropic vitamin.

A Committee of Longevity was formed in the U.S. in 1940. Its members are one-time students of the College of Physicians and Surgeons of Columbia University. Their object is to study disease prevention and the conditions necessary for lengthening the life span. The average age of members is in the seventies. Many are between 80 and 85. They are using every means known to medical science—including nutrition and endocrinology—to prove by their own example that health and life can be prolonged. Lately, membership has been extended to wives of members. If they were not made members, it was felt, the committee would come to consist largely of widowers.

In Russia, doctors and scientists have taken the subject of longevity very seriously for some time. One of the pioneers of the theory of rejuvenation was Metchnikov. He believed that old age is a disease and that its pre-mature appearance, according to scientific reckoning, was due to poisoning of the organism—self-poisoning or autointoxication. Other famous names in rejuvenation research are Metalnikov, Filatov, Lepeshinskaya, and Alexander and Victor Bogomoletz.

Professor Alexander Bogomoletz founded the Institute of Experimental Biology and Pathology of the Ukraine and was President of the Academy of Sciences of the Ukraine. He was celebrated for his theory that the secret of keeping young lay in the connective tissues; the "packaging" of our organs and tissues, which had not been given much attention before his researches.

The connective tissue, says Bogomoletz, is the chief factor in defending, preserving, and stimulating the human organism. According to him, we become old physically (and mentally also) because of changes in the connective tissue. The body is less and less able to absorb nourishment (under this heading water is included); in a sense, we die of starvation. Bogomoletz puts it this way: "The nutrition of the cells becomes disturbed, hunger follows, vital activity decreases; old age and death ensue."

His famous antireticular-cytotoxic serum (ACS for short) was evolved as an answer. It is a substance, he claimed, which becomes a factor in the stimulation and regeneration of the connective tissue and, through this medium, of the tissues and cells of the whole body.

The serum is said to be effective in the treatment of certain cancerous conditions; it is used, it seems, in many Soviet hospitals for many kinds of disease with excellent results. But the nature of the materials from which it is made, and the extreme difficulty of preparation, make it so rare outside Russia that, if we had to depend on ACS injections to keep us going, our chances of reaching 180 wouldn't be worth much.

Professor Alexander Bogomoletz' relative, Victor, developed a method of preventing and reversing the aging process that he called *Externotherapy*. This aims at stimulating and nourishing the connective tissue and the endocrine system (and, through them, the other cells of the body) by means of the skin. The skin, which is being recognized more and more by science as having a most important influence on the health, is prepared by Externotherapy's methods to absorb certain substances which act upon the cells of the body, reactivating its functioning.

"Tissular" therapy is the name given by another famous
Russian biologist, Professor Filatov, to his method of de-
laying and reversing the aging processes. His work was
based on his discovery that there are substances which—
when tissues decompose, are attacked, or are hurt in any
way—are produced in great quantities. They have tremendous energizing powers which are capable of regener-
ating living tissue. We have all seen, many times, the
action of these substances: decomposing tissue of dead
leaves, plants, or animals is the best fertilizer of new
growth. Perhaps Omar Khayyam had something when he
said:

"I sometimes think that never blows so red
   The rose, as where some buried Caesar bled . . ."

Filatov was apparently the first biologist to identify these
substances and to experiment with them. *Biogenic stimulins* he called them. They are not actually a substance, he
said, but a collection of substances whose composition has
not yet been determined. They are at least partially heat-
resistant; they keep their properties after having been
heated for one hour at a temperature above the boiling
point. They are soluble in water and can be distilled as
water vapor. They are neither an albumin nor a ferment.

Biogenic stimulins are present, Filatov discovered, in all
living tissues, from plant to man, and also in the soil itself.
The earth is a rich repository of these dynamic stimulins.
Filatov's theory is that the therapeutic value of water
springs is not explained solely by mineral salt content but
at least in part by the living substances, such as the stimu-

lins, with which they have become charged during their wanderings underground.

"Tissular" therapy is the harnessing of the power of these stimulins for human use. Filatov found that this could be done by introducing a very small piece of "dead" human tissue under the skin. This tissue worked through the connective tissue of the host, through the blood stream and all the cells, renewing them and their activities. The best form of foreign tissue for this purpose, Filatov discovered, was a segment of sterilized human placenta.

Tissular therapy is said to bring about a regeneration of the entire organism. Today this complete form of regeneration is realized as being the only sound method of tackling the "aging" problem. Earlier methods of hormone injections, grafts and the like affected one function or organ only. As a result, the balance of the glandular system might be upset. Reactions were not controlled. The danger of stimulating one set of glands or organs is realized much more clearly today than it was in the pioneering days of rejuvenation.

Professor Filatov insisted that any genuine rejuvenation or regeneration must come through influencing the energies of the entire organism. The Italian biologist Tallarico has said of these stimuli: "They make themselves felt on the organism as a whole . . . activating its vital potential and increasing its capacity for resistance, thus stimulating the power of healing and regeneration."

Dr. Victor Bogomoletz, I believe, has made use of the biogenic stimulins in conjunction with Externotherapy. The principles of the two methods are related, but the scope of Externotherapy is wider. It takes into consideration other factors besides the physical method of treatment. Dr. Bogomoletz believes that psychological and spiritual elements must also play an important part in total rejuvenation.

Since we have minds as well as bodies, this is only common sense. And I believe that the mind can prove an aid of tremendous power in the fight against premature death and decay. We must make use of it, and of the discoveries of science such as nutrition, the "basic factor," and of all methods which help mind and body to renew themselves.

It is a great adventure.

You may not realize how great it is until you feel response in your body to your efforts. But as you find yourself capable of more and more, instead of less and less, the horizons of life widen once more, beyond the few short years which were their narrow compass.

From now on, you can forget your age. Don't be hypnotized by what your birth certificate says. Chronological age doesn't matter. Biological age does—and you can begin to grow younger now, at this moment, if—as Dr. Börtz says— you will help yourself to do that.

Or do you feel that the infirmities, the ugliness, the disabilities of age are our lot and that from them there is no escape?

They are only inescapable if we accept them. Begin now to deny them. Never forget *old age is a disease, and it is curable*.

Now is the time to begin the cure.

CHAPTER

3

A SURVEY OF
THE PROGRAM

WE do not need to accept premature aging, with its difficulties, infirmities and indignities, as our fate. Nor premature death. "At eighty, we should not even be entering the prime of life." That was the considered opinion of the Berne Medical Congress recently held. Dr. Douglas Latto, the eminent London dietician and consultant, agrees with the findings of this conference on longevity. These are his actual words. "We have all the resources and researchers of chemistry, biochemistry, nutrition, biology, physiology, psychology, and parapsychology to help and support us—to enable us to reach our full span of life. We can live long without growing old."

You will remember that I quoted Dr. Christopherson of London Hospital as saying that a man "might live 300,

400, or even 1000 years, if the life-sustaining elements were present." Professor Starling mentions that recent discoveries about the chemistry of the body should make possible prolongation not of old age but of youth. Speaking of ways and means of conquering old age and decay, Dr. George Aldridge says that, as a result of biochemic discoveries, "life will be prolonged, the race will be made better and stronger, and many moral, spiritual, as well as material blessings will follow in its train."

"We can make old age wait," says Dr. Tom Spies. Those of us who succeed in doing so must obviously be fit in mind and body, a nucleus of a "better and stronger race."

Well, the potential is there. As we have seen, man is the only animal whose biologic clock does not run to its limit—seven to fourteen times the number of years in which individuals mature.

Biologic clocks run for periods (according to the species in which they operate) between a few hours and hundreds of years. The life cycle of some insects is a day; others live for a few months or a year. Then we have birds and animals which live up to about twenty years. And there are species whose members are mostly centenarians plus—birds, fish, and animals, among them carp, pike, eagles, parrots, crocodiles, and elephants.

There is the same variation in the setting of the biologic clocks in plant life, although so far there is no clue to its underlying cause. Some types of tree, such as the sequoias of California, live for thousands of years; others, oaks for instance, merely for hundreds. An oak tree at Catsfield, near Hastings, England, nearly reached the 1000 mark. It was there—probably not more than a sapling—when William the Conqueror landed in 1066. It has just been cut down because it was thought to be decaying. But it had managed to survive 900 years.

Even more inexplicable is the fact that some individuals of a species live two or three times as long as the rest of their relatives. There is the rose tree in Germany which has lived hundreds of years longer than the normal span of its kin; a cypress in Chapultepec, Mexico, is said to be 2000 years old. Cases of "centenarian" animals occur among their shorter-lived brethren. And in the days when general expectation of human life was much shorter than it is now, there were men and women who lived well toward their second century—such as Thomas Parr and the midwife of Charles I's queen.

Biologists think that the differing life span of species will be explained eventually by some "built-in" limiting factor. The individual "long-lifers" are Nature's darlings, they think. The body chemistry of these types is the perfect product.

Whatever the reason for these assorted lengths of survival, they show us that a life span can be extended almost indefinitely. And in the bee we have an example of what Nature herself does in that line. Worker bees and drones live four to five months. The queen bee can live about eight years.

The queen bee does not begin life as a super model. She comes from an ordinary egg and an ordinary larva. Her phenomenal life span (for a bee), her larger size and in general rather superior looks are the result of food.

All larvae in a hive get the same diet for their first three days. After that, only the larvae which are to become queens are specially fed. For the rest of their lives they eat only a substance called *royal jelly*. And it is this food, and this alone, which transforms ordinary larvae into queen bees.

But for us the answer is not quite so simple as for bees. We can't live in a controlled temperature on a specialized diet, with hundreds of attendants to wait on us, and follow a set pattern of existence. We have to overcome a number of threats to longevity; the "back-room boys" of biology have been investigating them. Apparently, senility is not among them. The percentage of people who die from true senility is a minute proportion of "old age" deaths.

Autointoxication (self-poisoning) is thought to be an arch-criminal as regards life-shortening. Unhealthy living conditions are a contributory factor. Lack of vitamins is another; and, says a London specialist, "Death is more frequently due to a lack of an adequately balanced supply of iron, copper, magnesium, and potassium than to any other cause."

The most high-powered killer of them all is thought to be the *stress syndrome*. This has been mentioned a good deal in the press and elsewhere in the last few years; it covers stress and strain of any kind. Worry, grief, fear, frustration—any emotions that make us tense and disturb us—upset the glandular mechanism of the body and digestion, increase blood pressure, and react adversely on every process and function. The stress syndrome breaks down the cells; it exhausts and destroys us. "We die because we think," if we allow ourselves continually to think negatively.

Mind over matter—the effect of mental states on the body—is getting a good deal of medical attention these days. The British cancer specialist Sir Heneage Ogilvie, mentioned elsewhere in this book, said he had never known a cancer patient without a mental problem. When there is anxiety of some kind, a difficulty which the mind cannot resolve, it turns it over, as it were, to the body. The problem objectifies itself as a headache or other ache, or illness of some kind. Some cases of asthma have been traced to unresolved difficulties and frustrations. The mechanism is in a way like that which causes an oyster to form a pearl around a foreign body of which it cannot rid itself. The basic irritation is hidden, but this is a make-shift measure, not a real solution.

The child—or adult—who wants to be the center of attention, and isn't, will often develop some physical ailment. The illness is "real," although its cause is in the mind. That is hardly surprising when one thinks how easily the body can be disturbed by the mind, and in particular how sensitive the glands are to its influence.

The functions of the body depend to a greater or lesser degree upon the functioning of the endocrine glands; if they are not working properly, there will soon be signs of ill health of some kind. Anything that affects one gland will eventually affect the others; although each gland has its own work to do, it is in very close association with the rest.

Each gland produces hormones which control or regulate physical processes. And in all this activity, the anterior lobe of the pituitary is the "king of the castle." In its turn, the pituitary gland is regulated by the nerve centers of the brain.

Here thought and emotion "pull the strings." And it is important to see that the stress syndrome is not pulling the wrong strings if we want to work against the onset of premature old age and death.

Before we begin this work, let us take a brief survey of the position and of the ways and means to be used in order to reach our goal.

THE FOOD FACTOR

Some nutritionists believe that by correct diet alone we ought to be able to increase our life span to normal—150 to 200 years. Correct diet means the right quantities of vitamins, minerals, protein, and the like, for the complex needs of the body. It does not mean food which only satisfies the feeling of hunger, which is no guide so far as real nutrition goes. The stomach is easily deceived temporarily. It would say "thank you very much" for a meal of old boot stewed till soft and tastily served. Correct diet means food in the sense of substances which satisfy the hidden hunger of the cells.

Food is a good starting point for our survey because it is the basic factor. Our bodies, our flesh and bones and blood, are made of the food we eat.

What we eat today walks and talks tomorrow. If our meals are poor from the real nutrition point of view—for instance if they are chiefly composed of white sugar, white flour, white bread, overcooked vegetables, not enough protein or fruit—the way we walk and talk will be affected.

The science of nutrition, the science of eating in fact, shows us that the way we eat has a powerful influence on health. Food deficiencies can cause disease; the right food can do a great deal to prevent it.

No doubt it can help us, also, a long way on the road towards our 180th birthdays. As we have seen, the life span of animals has been prolonged, doubled and even more, by planned diets containing the right amounts of the right foods. Symptoms of aging, graying fur, feebleness, and similar conditions have been reversed.

Real nutrition can work wonders with human beings, too. I would like to remind you of Dr. Tom Spies' work along these lines—the "resurrection" of 893 chronically ill people in Birmingham, Alabama, in particular. These people were in such a bad condition that they had not worked for years. The majority had been sent to the nutrition clinic after their own doctors had given them up as hopeless. Their treatment was correct diet, supplemented by massive doses of vitamins and minerals. These people recovered their health and were able to work again. Among them were shipbuilders, farm workers, miners— men who had to do a hard job of physical labor—as well as white-collar workers and housewives.

In England, some doctors (among them Harley Street men) are treating illnesses as *deficiency diseases*. One of these has had successes with cancer cases and with many forms of illness. Recently he was consulted by a woman who had had a form of diarrhea for nearly three months. Her own doctor had been able to do nothing for her; she had been to an orthodox specialist who could give her no treatment, and no hope. Progressively she was getting thinner and weaker. After three days of the deficiency-supplementation treatment, she improved. In a few weeks she was cured and there has been no relapse.

Let me quote, from my own experience, the case of a woman whose knees were as big as basketballs as a result of rheumatism. She could not bend them; she was never out of pain. She also had chronic skin irritation, periodic swelling of the face, weeping eczema on her fingers. Doctors and specialists told her there was no cure for any of these complaints; they said they did not know the cause. Planned eating, with diet supplements, put her right in a couple of months. When she went back to the hospital recently for a check-up, she was told: "You are cured. It's a miracle."

A woman who had hemorrhoids had been told the only cure was surgery, which she was reluctant to undergo. I suggested that she should try a planned diet and diet supplements, which she decided to do. In less than two months the hemorrhoids disappeared.

Often migraine yields to correct nutrition. I know several cases in which this has happened. And a scalp irritation which had been written off by doctors, treated in the same way, disappeared after a few weeks. It had been present for more than two years.

Dogs, too, can be helped by diet treatment. Paralysis, hysteria, skin troubles—all sorts of ailment can be due to food deficiencies. A partially paralyzed dachshund, which I treated by diet and mineral and vitamin supplements, recovered the use of its legs—although it had been condemned to death by the vet, who said he could do nothing. And a young dog, whose destruction also had been recommended because he had hysteria and fits, is now in the best of health and spirits after the same type of treatment.

These "miracles" of nutrition give some idea of what this new science is doing for us. As Sherman says, because of its researches we are better able to give our bodies what they need in order to keep young and healthy than ever before (at least in recorded history), because we know more of what those needs are.

The first step we must take toward lengthening our life span is to study the best ways of satifsying the "hunger of the cells." The cells in different parts of the body have different needs, but feeding them is not such a complicated business as it sounds.

You can draw up menus which reach the "real" nourishment standard without any difficulty from the lists given in later chapters of foods and the appendixes which contain the elements the cells must have. There is nothing out-of-the-way about the foods I have suggested. Eating for health simply means choosing foods which nourish the body and eliminating those which do not.

Diet will give you wonderful results. But although food is the basic factor, it is not the only one. Movement and the right use of the muscles can be sources of youth and health; the way we breathe is of paramount importance. And we cannot forget the part played by the dominant factor, the mind.

MOVEMENTS AND MUSCLES

Dr. Edward Börtz, a former president of the American Medical Association who believes that the normal span of our life should be at least 150, says that premature old age can be caused by muscles wasting away. Few people seem to realize this; and if they do, they do not realize that it need not happen—or that, even if it has happened, something can be done about it.

Flabbiness is Enemy No. 1 of youth; it is deterioration. To keep the body firm, the cells must be given the food elements they need to form healthy tissue; the muscles must be well fed. But they must also be used.

As we get older we tend to abuse, rather than to use, our muscles. We tend to underwork them—and that is as bad as overworking them. We are inclined to use legs, arms, hands, the whole body, in a half-hearted way and to let some muscles do work for which they were never intended. For instance, we use hands and arms to lever us up from a sitting position—work which should be done by the muscles of the thighs, abdomen, and diaphragm.

The less we ask of our muscles, the less they will do. So, by and by, we find that movement becomes effort instead of pleasure. Movement, when muscles are strong and coordinated, is a joy in itself. Everyone feels that joy when young: then we move for the sake of moving. And we lose it so gradually that we do not notice its going. We forget it, until it comes back again—until, well-fed and re-educated, the muscles begin to work once more as they were meant to work. Then, when we are in full control of our bodies again, we remember that we have not felt this way for years. In fact, we feel young!

The technique of muscle re-education is a most important part in our longevity program. One of the methods about which I shall tell you in a later chapter was used by the ancient Greeks during the peak period of their civilization, when their physical beauty was legendary.

BREATH

If we don't breathe, we don't live. We all know that is true. But what we don't all realize is that the better we breathe the better we live. The breath can be a source of energy and vitality and of health—if we breathe correctly. There is a great deal more in the way we breathe than we are apt to think. The rate and depth of inhalation and exhalation affects every function of the body, and influences the mind. A shallow, short breath is a life-shortener, we are told. And certainly animals whose breathing rate is more rapid than our own—dogs, for instance—live only about one quarter as long as we live. So our long-life program includes techniques for breathing longer—and deeper.

THE MIND

The mind, with its power of influencing the body for good or ill, cannot be left out of our calculations. Mental suggestion can produce far-reaching results on and changes in our physical system. The image-making faculty of the mind can speed up the results for which we are working. Another aspect of the mind's power is the stress syndrome and the havoc it can produce in the body. How are we to avoid being destroyed by the strain, the friction, the frustration with which we meet constantly?

A whole book could be written on this subject alone. At the present moment, we can deal only with its *ABC*s. And we can take comfort from the fact that just as the mind affects the body, so does the body affect the mind. So, by the use of controlled breathing and methods of rehabilitating the muscles and the whole physical mechanism, the mind becomes steadier and more controlled. Improving bodily health reacts on the mental condition and on the brain itself. The fact that movement has a reflex action on the brain has been proved by training mentally deficient children through motor culture. As a result, intellectual ability was improved.

So we have a line of defense against the stress syndrome.

And as we build up, brick by brick as it were, our own powers, we build up the ability to live out our normal life span in full health and activity.

That is our program.

SUMMARY

OUR PROGRAM for longevity has a simple motto and elements.

The motto, in the words of Dr. Tom Spies, is this:
We can make old age wait!

The elements, which we shall consider in detail throughout the rest of the book, are simple but vital. They are:
- Food
- Movement and the proper use of muscles
- Proper breathing
- The mind

CHAPTER

4

FOOD—THE BASIC FACTOR

EVERY activity of the mind and the body depends to a greater or lesser extent upon the food we eat; in that sense food is the basic factor of our lives, and nutrition is the basic science. The wrong food can be a destructive influence, causing illness and disease, affecting mental powers, shortening life. The right food can be a safeguard against bad health, can build us up on all levels, and—as we have seen—can make a powerful contribution toward long life and long youth.

Yet almost nothing is known about eating, generally; about eating in its real sense. And this always seems to be a blind spot in the human race. Would you turn a child, who knew only the *ABC*s of chemistry, loose in a laboratory stocked with powerful chemicals, some of them dangerous, and let him play about with them just as he fancied? He could, with no trouble at all, blow himself up, or burn or mutilate himself. He would be lucky to escape without some form of injury. Yet when most of us sit down to lunch or dinner, in our lack of knowledge of the effects on our system of what we are putting into our stomach we are very much in the same boat as the child in the laboratory. The effects of food chemicals may not be so spectacular or so immediate as those in the laboratory, but they are just as certain. They are governed by the laws of biochemistry.

The commonsense thing, you would think, would be to have the elementary facts of nutrition taught in all schools —and what a difference we should see in the national health in a generation, if this were done. And centers where these facts were available could be established in almost every town and village. At any rate, some way should be found of getting across vital, practical information about the right use of food to adults, men as well as women. And it should be found without delay, before the standard of national health drops any lower. People constantly ask me why no such places exist; it is one of my dreams to see such centers come into being—centers where people could be shown the vital relationship between food and health and youth and long life—where mothers would discover why Mary can't eat eggs, or Harold doesn't like sugar. Childish likes and dislikes of certain foods may seem trivial, but often they are valuable clues to the body's workings. These can be followed up, used to safeguard health, to improve "difficult" characters (which often are a result of dietary deficiencies), and even make schoolwork easier by increasing mental ability and aiding memory.

To bring all this about, the average person need not get bogged down in a mass of complicated detail; it would be enough to know the broad principles of nutrition. After all, we have to learn something about mathematics so that we can cope with everyday affairs, but we don't have to be Einsteins.

The next time you are in a bus or train, or even reading a newspaper, look at the advertisements, and you will see what I mean about the national health standard. I haven't actually worked out the proportion of different types of advertisement, but I think there's no doubt that those concerned with remedies for illness of some kind are way ahead numerically of the others. Headaches, colds, coughs, fatigue, constipation, indigestion—wherever we go, we can't escape from reminders that most of us splutter, wheeze, and hiccup our way through life, and stumble along racked by rheumatism or arthritis.

Food is not a panacea for all this: don't misunderstand me as saying that. But it is the *basic* factor, and we should give it the attention which is its due.

STARTING-POST

At the beginning of the track which leads to our 180th birthdays, the starting-post is the *balanced meal*. Before doing anything else, we must get into the habit of balancing our meals. That means every menu should include protein (meat, cheese, eggs, fish), carbohydrate (sugar, starch), fat, and an adequate supply of vitamins and minerals. I will discuss these two items in greater detail later on. Fruit and vegetables must be eaten at each meal, not only for their vitamins and minerals, but because they are mainly alkaline-forming foods, necessary to preserve the alkaline-acid balance in the blood.

You may have noticed that I haven't mentioned between-meal snacks or tea as meals. This is because they shouldn't be meals. Bread and butter, sandwiches (anyone who has read *Eat and Stay Young* will know my opinion of sandwiches, at any time, in any place), cakes, at teatime or otherwise, are just an unnecessary chore for the system to cope with. Washing down all that carbohydrate with tea doesn't help, either; it lessens the stomach's ability to cope with a mass of excess starch. Carbohydrate is the one dietary item you can be sure most people are not short of; we all tend to eat too much starch. And, especially as we grow older, we cannot afford to do so. We should cut down ruthlessly on starches, for the sake of health as well as looks.

Everyone needs *some* starch in the diet, of course, and the amount varies with the individual. The governing factor is the way each individual's body works; the rate of metabolism varies a little with everyone. But the amount of starch in the average diet is unbelievable, and out of all proportion to the body's needs. Here are some examples.

BREAKFAST

Even people who say they don't eat breakfast will have a couple of slices of toast or so, with jam or marmalade (in which there is sugar), and perhaps a breakfast cereal with sugar. *And* probably sugar in their coffee. Admitted breakfast eaters probably have cereal with sugar, maybe sometimes fried bread with their protein dish of eggs and bacon or poached eggs on toast, plus a few slices of toast and marmalade.

MID-MORNING

The average coffee break is cruelty to stomachs—cakes, cookies, sweetened coffee or tea, most likely. Or a sandwich.

LUNCH

Perhaps thick soup (made with flour), potatoes with the main dish *and* bread, and something else made with flour, whether it's elaborate pastry or just a cake. Possibly sweetened tea or coffee again.

TEA OR COFFEE BREAK

See above.

DINNER

Could be thick soup again, bread *and* potatoes with main dish, a pudding-type dish made with flour as for lunch, or perhaps a savory such as macaroni and cheese, often plus potatoes, and no green vegetables. Perhaps cheese *and* crackers afterward or pie or cake and sweetened coffee.

AT BEDTIME

Often cookies are nibbled, adding to the quota which all too often is downed during the day between meals.

I think you will agree that the amount of starchy items on the menu I have quoted is not exaggerated. Perhaps your starch ration is lower than this, but I am sure you know many people who eat carbohydrate at every meal, and a great deal of it. Generally, it is in the form of white flour, white sugar, and white bread, which means that the minerals and vitamins—whose function it is to help the system to deal with starch—are reduced or absent. Consistently overloading the body with any kind of food it doesn't need has a result something like stopping up a sink. The waste-disposal mechanism has more than it can deal with; substances which should have been cleared away deteriorate and produce a poisonous condition—autointoxication. This is a cordial invitation to many kinds of ills, not excluding the very-common cold.

So starch and sugar, or at least too much of them, are enemies of long life and youth, and must be used only in their right proportion to other foods. Here is a guide as to how that can be done.

BREAKFAST

An egg, or kidney (grilled), or bacon (grilled), or fish (not fried); not more than a total of two slices of whole-meal bread, butter, honey. Fresh fruit. No cereal.

MID-MORNING

Milk drink of some kind. No cookies, cakes, or sandwiches.

LUNCH

Clear soup, tomato juice, or fresh fruit juice, if desired. Meat, fish, cheese, egg (if not eaten at breakfast); potato (two small or one large) cooked in the skin, *or* one slice whole-meal bread with butter. Green vegetables or salad. Fresh fruit.

AFTERNOON

Weak *café au lait* or weak tea. No cakes, cookies, bread.

EVENING MEAL

Same as at lunchtime.

In passing, here are one or two points worth remembering when choosing items on your menu. The easiest way to make sure you are getting full benefit from meat, fish, cheese, and related foods (the protein part of the meal) is to have some form of protein at each meal: an egg at breakfast; meat, cheese, or fish at lunch and the same in the evening. It isn't a good plan to miss protein at one meal and say to yourself you'll eat a double ration at the next meal.

It isn't a good plan because it isn't the body's plan, and the body always has the last word on the subject. It will not use large amounts of protein in a lump, so to speak; excess of its needs at any one time will be excreted. The golden rule for eating protein for maximum benefit is to have a more or less regular amount at more or less regular intervals.

Another golden rule is always to eat a small amount of starch food, such as bread or potatoes, with protein. Otherwise some of the protein will be burned as energy—which is a wasteful way of getting energy, since the purpose of protein is the vital purpose of building, maintaining, and repairing the cells; and the formation of antibodies, which attack germs of disease, and hormones, which are necessary for organic action.

Young people need plenty of good fresh meat, fish, eggs, and cheese for their growing bodies; adults also need this form of food in order to keep going. Once it was thought that old people did not need much of it, but now it has been found that they do, and the standard of health in older people has improved accordingly.

Food variety is essential to health. Most foods have different vitamins and minerals in them, all necessary to important physical processes. There are twenty amino-acids in proteins, of which at least ten must be "among those present" in our daily diet. It is thought that we are able to synthesize—to produce in our internal chemical factories—the other amino-acids.

Different kinds of meat, fish, cheese, and other protein foods are composed of different amino-acids (which are linked in proteins rather as paper chains are linked), so the more you can vary your meals the better, in order to include all the amino-acids in your food.

Some proteins have a better food value (or what is called *biologic value*) than others, because their "chains" are made up in much the same way as the protein chains of the human body are made. Meat, eggs, and cheese are the best choices from this point of view. The protein of fish isn't so good as that of meat; milk is on the poor side for an adult's needs; the protein of leguminous vegetables, such as beans and peas, and of nuts, is not easily made use of by the human body.

However, when two proteins which by themselves would not be worth a great deal in food value are eaten together, our "inside chemistry" gets to work and produces a useful protein from two second-class ingredients. For instance, whole-grain cereal combined with milk, or nuts with whole-meal bread, would be quite well utilized for protein requirements.

It really isn't necessary for most of us to memorize the names of the essential amino-acids, and to go around worrying about whether we have had our isoleucine or our tryptophane today, so long as we make every effort to vary the menu as often as we can, and to see that protein of high biologic value figures on it. Those, as I said, are the important points to keep in mind.

The same principle applies to the minerals which we must have in order to keep on the health standard—to say nothing of keeping our youth. There are ninety-two known mineral elements. A number of them have been found in the human body tissues; many in microscopic amounts, to which the name *trace* or oligo elements has been given. Scientists think that all the minerals are present, or should be, in our bodies, although perhaps in such infinitesimal quantities that as yet we have no instruments delicate enough to register them. In the meantime, they may be tracked down by induction—much as an astronomer gets clues to the existence of some planet or star.

The trace elements act mostly as co-workers with the major elements, and as catalyzers. A *catalyzer* is a substance which speeds a process. A well-known definition of catalytic action is that it is like a tip to a waiter—it accelerates a reaction which would otherwise proceed with infinite slowness.

Minerals also work together in chains, each link of which depends for efficiency on the rest. For instance, one such chain consists of vanadium, manganese, iron, cobalt, nickel, copper, and zinc. A deficiency of any one of these elements can be the underlying cause, chemically speaking, of anemia. In plants, the deficiency will cause a similar condition, but in plants it is called chlorosis.

The whole gamut of physical existence, from the soil to man, is dependent upon minerals for health. The great nutritionist Professor Sherman is among those who believe that minerals, in particular calcium, are essential to longevity. The life span of laboratory animals has been increased enormously by increasing the amount of calcium in their diet.

Although our daily quota of minerals is all-important, we need not, as I said a few paragraphs back, carry out chemical analyses to discover how much nickel there may be in mussels, or how much potassium is present in potatoes. A balanced diet, as widely varied as possible, with plenty of fresh fruit and vegetables, is the answer; it will keep our cells healthy and happy.

But even in what seems an ideal diet, there are pitfalls. Not all fresh fruit and vegetables are equally useful. Spinach, for instance, converts calcium in the body into a useless mass; so do other plants of the goosefoot family. Rhubarb has the same effect. Plums and prunes disturb the mineral balance of the body. I would advise eating these food items seldom and sparingly; children are better off without them, at least until they are in their late teens. Beware of uncooked white of egg; it contains a substance called avidin, which inactivates one of the B vitamins, biotin. Cooking puts avidin out of action; it also reduces the phytic acid in whole-grain cereals, which otherwise would make useless some of the body's calcium.

The points I have just mentioned are examples of vital items of food knowledge, which I urge should be taught in all schools and emphasized at nutrition information centers. They may sound small matters only, but one cannot dismiss a fact as insignificant because it is small. You remember the verse that begins "For the want of a nail, the shoe was lost"—and ends with the loss of a kingdom? These small dietary points merit careful attention, want of which could cause eventually enough calcium to be lost from, say, a child's body to be disastrous. In the end, a life might be lost. And it is worth remembering that nervousness and many other manifestations of neuroticism are due to calcium deficiency.

In general, a very great deal of ill health, physical and mental, and many serious diseases might be avoided if little details about the "basic factor" were more widely known.

SUMMARY

FOOD IS THE BASIC FACTOR in our program for long life and long youth. The starting point in assuring proper food is a *balanced diet,* as widely varied as possible.

Every meal should include
- protein (meat, cheese, eggs, fish)
- carbohydrate (sugar, starch)
- fat
- vitamins and minerals
- fruit and vegetables

Here are sample meals for one day that will afford balance and variety
- **Breakfast:** an egg, grilled kidney or grilled bacon, or fish (not fried); not more than two slices of whole-meal bread; butter and honey. Fresh fruit. No cereal.

- **Morning and afternoon food breaks:** Milk drink of some kind in the morning; weak milky coffee or weak tea in the afternoon. No cookies, cakes, or sandwiches.
- **Lunch:** clear soup, tomato juice, or fresh fruit juice. Meat, fish, cheese, egg (if none eaten at breakfast); one large or two small potatoes cooked in the skin—or one slice whole-meal bread with butter. Green vegetables or salad. Fresh fruit.
- **Dinner:** same as lunch.

A few foods to avoid

- Spinach and rhubarb—convert calcium in the body into a useless mass
- Plums and prunes—also disturb the mineral balance
- Uncooked white of egg—contains a substance that inactivates biotin, one of the useful B vitamins

CHAPTER

5

FUEL FOR GLANDS

Y OUR GLANDS influence every part of your body.

Can you influence your glands? Can you help or hinder their all-important functions? I think the answer is that you can, by quite natural means. By providing them with ample and regular supplies of the food materials they must have and by forms of exercise which ensure that the blood flows to them as it should flow, you can make it possible for your glands to stay young and to continue to function vigorously.

Treatment of the glands with drugs and hormonal injections and grafts by Voronoff, Steinach, and others produced results, as we have been told. There was an appearance of rejuvenation, but it did not last. The rejuvenation was not truly effective. And, when the effects of the treatment wore off, there was a relapse. So far at least, it seems

46

that we cannot hope to improve the condition and action of the glands by such means.

Scientists tell us that it is not in the body's best interest to try to rejuvenate merely one gland. No part of the body is an independent unit; each is dependent to some extent upon the other parts. Overstimulation in one direction can lead to disturbance in others, rather as if one were to speed up enormously the action of one part of the machinery of a watch without considering the effect upon the rest of the works.

Some of the modern pioneers of rejuvenation seem to have used the specialized rejuvenation technique. The sex glands got most of the attention—the theory being, roughly speaking, that these glands are sources of vital energy, that rejuvenation of the gonads would result in restoring youth to the whole body.

It was a good idea, but it didn't work. It has been found that the aging of the human system is not caused by the weakening of the sex glands alone—though, of course, the decline in sexual function may be a symptom that the aging processes have begun. Not only do the gonads (sex glands) deteriorate, but also the entire endocrine system, though even this is believed to be not a cause but an effect of aging. The direct, immediate cause, say biologists, is the changes taking place in the connective tissue.

And the cause of these changes? In the last analysis, scientists tell us, the cause lies in the mind. Dr. Alexander Bogomoletz says: "The prolonged youth and long life of our body chiefly depends on the condition of our mind [or psyche]. . . ."

Remember that phrase. It is worth taking note of; it

is a vital clue to the problems of longevity. We shall come back to this point later.

Sexual life itself is not dependent solely on the organic state of the glands. Psychological influences are as important as physical factors to its functioning. As Bogomoletz says, "We must cease to consider the sexual problem as a strictly glandular problem."

Not even the mighty pituitary itself has the last word, you will remember. The pituitary is controlled by the brain.

This fact and its inferences bring us to the fringe of new country; it is the beginning of journeys to unknown destinations. Four hundred years ago, when Elizabeth I was queen of England, the physical world was giving up its secrets to our ancestors. Our explorations today are of a different character, but they may have a more profound effect on our destinies.

In the meantime, what can we do about our glands? The effects upon them of the application of psychological influences will be considered later. First, let us see what can be done with the basic factor, food, to improve their condition and functioning.

The possibilities are promising.

Food, obviously, is the raw material out of which are made the secretions of the glands and from which the tissues of the glands themselves are renewed. Food can stimulate the glands to produce hormones or it can have the effect of reducing the output.

Every time we eat, we set going a chain of causes which affects the glands and—of course—eventually every atom of our bodies. That realization does not mean that we should turn into food-fussers, but it does mean that in order to get the glands to do what we want, we must give them what *they* want, which is only common sense. So now let us see what raw materials we need in order to build up glands which will last for 180 years or more. First comes the needs of the pituitary.

THE PITUITARY GLAND

This gland, situated roughly behind the nose, at the base of the brain, is really two glands, anterior and post-pituitary. The anterior pituitary is connected with growth and with sexual development. The post-pituitary is the regulating factor of the water balance of the body, of the blood pressure. It influences the workings of the digestive and sex organs. It is related to skin coloring and to the complexion; it also affects the metabolism of sugar and fat in the system. Very important work—and all done by a mere speck of body substance, weighing six-tenths of a gram.

PITUITARY NEEDS

First, an adequate supply of water. This is vital to keep the post-pituitary in good condition. The vital vitamin is B. Deficiency of this vitamin has been found to cause deterioration of the pituitary, which in turn affects the sex functions, among others. The damage to men is much greater than to women, because lack of Vitamin B causes a form of degeneration of the testes, but not of the ovaries. Vitamin E is also important; more Vitamin E is found in the post-pituitary than in any other gland. Manganese is the mineral most necessary to the health of the post-pituitary.

Food Sources of Vitamin B

Wheat germ (which also contains Vitamin E), yogurt, black molasses, whole-grain cereals, brewers' yeast.

Food Sources of Manganese

Potatoes, lettuce (which also contains Vitamin E), wheat germ, walnuts and almonds, liver, peanuts, agar-agar (a seaweed product), raw egg-yolk, parsley, olives. The pituitary, and indeed all the glands, need abundant protein for healthy functioning.

THYROID GLAND

Situated in the throat, astride the windpipe and near the larynx, the thyroid is the "pep" gland. When it is working as it should, it makes you feel you can take on the world —and all comers. The thyroid gives us the magnetism of vitality and *joie de vivre*. On it, to a great extent, depends the way we look. It keeps the nails, the hair, and the complexion healthy and in good condition. Deficiency of the secretion of the thyroid, thyroxin, makes us tired, our flesh soft and flabby, and our minds lazy. We forget easily, can't register quickly, and have cold feet, actually and metaphorically. An inactive thyroid is apt to make us fat —and lazy. A thyroid-deficient type crawls around as if he doesn't much want to get where he is going; the owner of a normally functioning thyroid strides along as if he were on his way to collect a fortune.

A weak thyroid affects the sex glands, causing apathy and loss of interest in that aspect of life. Extreme thyroid deficiency is indicated by the appearance of goiter. A healthy thyroid is an important youth factor. Removal or malfunctioning of this gland can produce symptoms of age in a young person in a relatively short time.

THYROID NEEDS

Iodine is a prerequisite. On it the working of the thyroid largely depends. A constant supply of iodine is essential in order to keep up the supply of thyroxin in the blood. We have already seen what happens when it isn't there.

Vitamin B (the whole of the B group or complex) is also essential to thyroid health, as is Vitamin C. Vitamin C is a "must" because it is necessary for effective absorption of one of the amino-acids, tyrosine. (For food sources of Vitamin B see list under PITUITARY, above, and in the Appendix.)

Tyrosine is one of the amino-acids from which some proteins are formed. It has been found that tyrosine is just as necessary to the thyroid as is iodine; in other words, it is a "must."

Food Sources of Iodine

Seafood, particularly oysters, shrimps, salmon; cod-liver oil, watercress, tomatoes, radishes, dark berries, beetroot, asparagus, Irish moss (dried carageen), and all sea-greens. These latter should be eaten in some form every day. They can be bought in powder form, from which jellies and aspics, blancmanges, and so on can be made. They can also be used for thickening soups and gravies, and are better for this purpose than the usual thickening agents.

Food Sources of Vitamin C

Black currants, rose-hips, lemons, oranges, tomatoes, cabbage,* turnip-tops, almost all fresh vegetables and fruit.

Food Sources of Tyrosine

It is to be found in most proteins, particularly in casein, one of the proteins of milk. It is a close chemical relation of thyroxin, the secretion of the thyroid, and of melanin, the pigment substance. Tyrosine is one of the essentials in preventing gray hair and in helping to restore the hairs original color. Vitamin C, as we have seen, must be present for its effective use by the system.

GONADS (SEX GLANDS)

These glands are important for general health and well-being as well as for the sex functions. They not only produce external secretions (potential offspring), but also internal secretions which pass into the blood stream and have a revitalizing effect on the system. They are easily affected by lack of essential elements which are present in certain foods; a great deal of sterility and loss of virility can be traced to dietary deficiencies. Actually, a normal sex life can be continued up to what is considered by present standards an advanced age. The extension of our active life span would be the extension of all our functions. Plato tells us that the Pelasgians kept the color of

* Cabbage increases the need for iodine, as does liver. Butter and cod-liver oil are "iodine sparing."

their hair (active thyroid), their eyesight, and their virility to the end of their lives—200 years or so.

THE GONADS' NEEDS

Vitamins A, B, C, and E. Vitamin A is essential for the health of the ovaries and for the prostate. Prostate trouble could no doubt be avoided in many cases by a sufficiency of Vitamin A in the diet. This vitamin also controls the sexual cycle. Vitamins of the B group are important for maintaining libido and virility. You remember that this vitamin complex is vital for the pituitary gland's health, which has such a potent influence on the sex functions. These things all tie up together. Vitamin C is particularly essential for the ovaries; its deficiency can produce in either sex a kind of anemia (among other results) which damages the gonads.

Vitamin E has been labeled the fertility vitamin. Its deficiency causes sterility in both sexes. In the male, lack of Vitamin E first affects sperm production, then the fertility of the sperm, and finally causes complete lack of sex interest.

Deficiency of the B vitamins usually is accompanied by anxiety and general feelings of frustration or worry. As the deficiency usually reduces the ability to function normally sexually, a vicious circle is set up. Fortunately, when the missing links in the diet are supplied, the symptoms disappear, unless, of course, the condition has been allowed to go on so long that the damage is irreversible.

Protein

None of the glands can get along without a proper supply of protein. A high-protein diet is absolutely essential to the proper functioning of the sex glands. Starvation diets quickly and completely kill sex interest; animals on inadequate protein food do not mate. Arginine (one of the amino-acids) is thought to be important, in particular, to the action of these glands.

Minerals

Iron and copper. Copper is essential for assimilation of iron in the system.

Food Sources of Vitamin A

Fish-liver oil, potatoes, kale, broccoli, turnip greens, lettuce, apricots, carrots, peaches, prunes, tomatoes, kidneys. (For food sources of Vitamins B and C, see previous lists and complete list in the Appendix.)

Food Sources of Vitamin E

Wheat germ, wheat-germ oil, lettuce, avocado pears, egg-yolk, whole-grain cereals, sunflower-seed oil.

Food Sources of Arginine

Eggs, milk, oatmeal, peanut flour, whole wheat, yeast, and many other proteins. Let me repeat that arginine is an amino-acid, which is to be found in at least one of the proteins contained in eggs and milk. Every protein type of food contains several different kinds of protein. For instance, casein and lactalbumin are two proteins found in milk.

Food Sources of Iron

Lima beans, peas, whole wheat, oatmeal, raisins, eggs, green vegetables. The iron in meat is not easily available to the human body. Spinach is best forgotten as a source of iron, for reasons already mentioned.

Food Sources of Copper

Wheat germ, lentils, barley, liver, kidney beans, parsley, black molasses, mushrooms, asparagus.

ADRENALS

There are two of these small glands, about the size of the average man's thumb, perched on top of each kidney. They really are not two glands, but four; each adrenal is a double gland, consisting of an outer gland or cortex, and an inner gland or medulla. Each of these glands-within-a-gland produces a distinctive secretion which has its own job to do. These glands have been called the glands of combat and the glands of survival. The hormones they release into the blood stream enable us to fight if we must and, if we don't fight, to get away quickly enough to live to fight another day.

The secretion of the cortex controls brain growth and the development of the sex glands, and helps to maintain their healthy condition after adolescence. It also regulates the acid level of the body.

The adrenals are concerned in protein metabolism. And it is thought that one cause of graying hair could be that the adrenals were not working properly. A deficiency of one of the secretions of the adrenals, adrenalin, slows up reactions. These glands are one of our defenses against toxins in the body, which they are able to destroy.

These glands are very sensitive to shortage of the elements they need in food. Chemicals damage them easily; lead and nicotine are particularly dangerous to them.

ADRENALS' NEEDS

High-protein diet—of course. Vitamins A, E, and perhaps particularly C are necessary to their efficient working. As with the thyroid gland, proteins containing the amino-acid tyrosine should be regularly on the menu. (For food sources of Vitamins A, B, and C and tyrosine, see previous lists and the Appendix.)

PARATHYROID GLANDS

These important little glands are four in number, and have a total weight of only about half a gram. They are so close to the thyroid glands, in the throat, that until about fifty years ago they were thought to be part of the thyroid. Their chief function is to regulate our calcium supply. They dole it out where it is most needed; they mobilize it from the body's calcium hoard in the bones, the trabeculae, in time of shortage. And since calcium is the mainstay of the nerves, parathyroid deficiency shows itself, as you would expect, in great sensitivity of the nervous system, uncontrollable irritation—what is generally known as "temperament" when we want to be polite. Reduced calcium level in the blood produces allergies, cramps, and spasms.

PARATHYROID NEEDS

The vital factor is Vitamin D, which enables the system to take up calcium, regulates the calcium-phosphorus balance in the body, exercises a stabilizing influence on the parathyroids themselves, and is thought to act through them. A plentiful supply of calcium is necessary to keep these glands in good condition.

Food Sources of Vitamin D

Few foods contain Vitamin D. The best sources are egg-yolk, fatty fish, and fish-liver oils. Since in the winter months less Vitamin D is present in most foods, it is best to take cod-liver oil or halibut-liver oil as a food supplement. The action of the sun on the skin enables our bodies to synthesize the vitamin, so in summer deficiencies of this vitamin are less likely.

Food Sources of Calcium

This mineral is top-ranking in importance to health and youth. Many authorities think that most of us do not get enough of it in our food. The best sources are milk, cheese, oranges, apples, cabbage, cucumber, lettuce, radishes, watercress, whole wheat, carrots, beetroot—and honey.

THYMUS GLAND

The thymus gland is a neighbor of the heart. Its name comes from the Greek word *thumos,* which means heart—and also courage. The thymus is at its most active during childhood; at one time it was thought that as we became older this gland had little or no importance. But it has been found that, although it is less powerful in adolescence and in maturity, the thymus gland goes on functioning throughout life, even into old age. There is evidence that the thymus is related to growth, nutrition, and to the lymph cells in the blood. Vitamin B is the vital food factor. (For food sources of Vitamin B, see previous lists and the Appendix.)

PANCREAS

This is a large gland, as glands go. There are several inches of it lying across the abdominal cavity. Its secretion, insulin, which is produced in cells called the Islets of Langerhans, is a household word because of its association with diabetes. The other hormone it produces, kalikrein, is less well known, and no relationship between this hormone and food has been proved.

The pancreas is the sugar-controller of the system. Excessive amounts of sugar and fat on the menu eventually damage the pancreas through overwork. The usual result of such a breakdown is diabetes.

NEEDS OF THE PANCREAS

Vitamin B, which helps in the formation of insulin. Sulphur is of value, as are the amino-acids cystine and glutamic acid. Nickel is an essential mineral. (For food sources of Vitamin B, see previous lists and the Appendix.)

Food Sources of Cystine and Glutamic Acid

These are found in most proteins. Glutamic acid makes up more than 30 per cent of one of the proteins of milk (lactalbumin). This amino-acid is the chief factor of one of the enzymes of the brain. Plenty of glutamic acid in the diet helps the memory and strengthens the faculties of the mind.

Food Sources of Sulphur

Brussels sprouts, cauliflower, cabbage, lettuce, strawberries, gooseberries, egg-yolk, turnips, onions, coconut, carrots.

Food Sources of Nickel

Most vegetables and animal tissues.

Now you have an *ABC* of the glands and the foods which are vital to their health and youth—and to the whole body's wellbeing. Every day, at every meal, some of these foods should figure on the menu. It is an essential part of our program to make and keep the glands in good condition.

We know that the glands are key centers of health and youth. And we know that we can help them maintain their tone by the right food. A rich supply of blood is also essential to gland health. At the beginning of this chapter I mentioned certain forms of exercise which ensure that the blood flows to the glands as it should. These movements, or exercises, are described later in this book.

Another point which we must consider is that the glands are very sensitive to focused attention. If you will concentrate on each gland, or pair of glands, in turn, imagining and saying to yourself that each is working perfectly, you will find that their functioning is improved a great deal. This form of concentration must be carried out regularly, every day. It need take only a few minutes; you could

practice it when you wake in the morning, before getting
out of bed.

SUMMARY

THE GLANDS influence every part of the body. In turn, they
are controlled to a great extent by the mind and affected
by the supply of blood they get—factors that are explored
in later chapters. This chapter has discussed in detail the
basic factor, food, and indicated the raw materials the
glands need for good condition and best functioning.

Remember: *all glands need abundant protein for healthy
functioning.*

Here is a list of the nutritional needs of the body's glands.
For the food sources of each, see the Appendix.

- Pituitary needs
    Water
    Vitamin B
    Vitamin E
    Manganese
- Thyroid needs
    Iodine
    Vitamin B
    Vitamin C
    Tyrosine
- Gonads (sex glands) need
    Vitamins A, B, C, E
    Arginine
    Iron

Copper
- Adrenals need
    Vitamin C
    Vitamins A, E
    Tyrosine
- Parathyroids need
    Vitamin D
    Calcium
- Thymus needs
    Vitamin B
- Pancreas needs
    Vitamin B
    Sulphur
    Cystine and glutamic acid
    Nickel

CHAPTER

FATS CAN BE FATAL

Too much of the wrong kind of fat in your diet, not enough of the right kind—and your chances of reaching your 80th birthday, let alone your 180th, are slim.

According to modern medical reckoning, the fat we mostly eat either does not contain or has been robbed of substances which are necessary to the body. The vitamins which enable the fat-processing mechanisms to work are removed from bread and other foods. And chiefly for this reason, killer diseases, such as diseases of the arteries, are becoming a kind of twentieth-century Black Death.

From the aspect of diet we are discussing, there are two types of fat; one containing saturated fatty acids, which to all intents and purposes are antivitamins; the other containing what are called unsaturated fatty acids, or Vitamin F. The last-mentioned is the "right" type of fat, and is necessary to our 180 years. The others are the wrong type.

This chapter has a special message for men. It isn't for men only, however; it's very important for women also. But for some reason that has not yet been discovered, the male animal needs about five times more unsaturated fatty acids to keep him going than a woman needs. And as this is thought to be the reason why so many more men than women develop and die from coronaries, men should take a very special interest in Vitamin F.

The essential fatty acids (EFA for short) are rather like the amino-acids, which are the units that build up a protein substance. Essential fatty acids are units of fatty substance, such as olive oil, but they are not found in all types of fat. The fats which do not contain Vitamin F can be put into the "wrong" fat category. Broadly speaking, they are the "commercial" fats; fats which have been subjected to a hardening process so that they are easy to sell and to handle. And will keep. Distrust any food item which will keep for a long time: it is dead.

Margarine and shortenings of the types used in cooking, for frying, and so on, are examples. Most of them are made from excellent ingredients—vegetable oils or whale oil, which are rich in EFA. But the oils are hardened by hydrogenation, which destroys Vitamin F.

The "right" fats are built up with units of EFA and are not subjected to any process which would destroy their activity. Many animal oils, such as those of butter, egg-yolk, and lard, contain EFA, but it is not a good idea to let these loose, so to speak, in the diet because they have a high cholesterol content. Vegetable oils are cholesterol-free, but even these should be taken with discretion because the system will not cope with too much of anything.

Also, it can and will manufacture cholesterol from any kind of fat.

Olive oil, cottonseed oil, sunflower-seed oil, linseed oil, and soya-bean oil are good sources of EFA, and perhaps in some ways the best is wheat-germ oil, because it contains a high percentage of Vitamin E, an important factor in enabling the system to get the maximum results from EFA. Vitamin B_6 (pyridoxine) is also vital to the processing of EFA in the system.

Both these vitamins, E and B_6, are found in whole-meal bread and flour, which also contains wheat-germ oil. All the goods in one parcel, ready for use. This is the kind of planning followed out in nature's arrangements—the type of vitamin and the kind of mineral found in certain foodstuffs isn't just chance. The substances are there together because they belong together in the nutrition pattern.

But that is a fact which so many scientists will not grasp. They seem to think that they can go one better. In the case of bread and flour, which we are now discussing, the whole-meal articles are turned into white bread and flour, a process which demineralizes them, removes their unsaturated fatty acids and their vital vitamins, E and B.

Any lingering traces of these substances are wiped up by the addition of enriching agents—so called. I can think of more suitable names for them. These are chemical substances which are supposed to be harmless, from a toxic point of view. But no one knows what far-reaching effects they may have in disturbing the delicate chemistry of the body; effects which could only be recognized by experts over a period of years. Other additions are made to the dough during baking: glyceryl monostearate, stearyl tartrate, polyoxyethylene stearate. Nothing is known so far of the changes these chemicals produce in the action of EFA.

And after all, the result of the adding and subtracting is what could be called artificial bread and flour, reconstituted and changed till they have only a slight resemblance to the originals. These artificial products constitute a danger to EFA, while the originals make a useful contribution to the body's EFA needs.

The body must have reasonable amounts of unsaturated fatty acids. Without them it cannot cope with cholesterol. Overloading of the system with cholesterol can cause "furring-up" of the arteries. The addition of EFA to the diet has been shown to lower serum cholesterol in man.

A great deal of research on this subject has been done and is still going on; one of the conclusions is that, although fat consumption has gone up, most people's food is lacking in EFA, for the reasons we have mentioned.

So there is a double-barreled threat now: excess of "danger" fat and lack of the materials necessary to dispose of it. Excess fat aggravates the Vitamin F deficiency, because it increases the demands of the system for that vitamin; lack of EFA increases the danger from unsaturated fats, which are liable to form abnormal combinations with cholesterol.

Such threats to long life and health as these must be considered so that we can avoid them.

EFA deficiency shows itself in a number of ways. Dr. J. E. Nirop, writing in the *Lancet,* believes that deficiency of EFA contributes to bronchial carcinoma, because the deficiency increases the sensitiveness of the system to a chemical substance in, for instance, tobacco, which can be cancer-producing. In general it is believed that an EFA deficiency makes us more sensitive to a number of substances known as *carcinogens* or potential cancer-causers. It is even possible that the sensitivity may be as great a danger as the carcinogen. A doctor once put it this way to me: "Almost anything *can* cause cancer, given the predisposition; a glass eye, a wooden leg, or false teeth—anything or any substance which causes irritation."

Men are particularly susceptible to cancer of the stomach. Some doctors think this may be explained by their sensitivity, due to Vitamin F deficiency, to chemical substances, which may be carinogenic, in processed foods. Men, you will remember, are more susceptible to this deficiency than are women because they need five times as much EFA.

The skin suffers from lack of EFA. There is a form of eczema, chiefly found in men, cases of which appear to be increasing. It is a complaint very similar to a skin trouble developed by rats deficient in EFA. The dermatitis which use of detergents causes in many people could, it is thought, be due to the removal of EFA by the chemical substances in the washing powders.

It is believed that a basic cause of these troubles is that a deficiency of EFA affects the structure of the skin. In certain experiments on animals lacking in EFA, the skin was found to show a remarkable increase in permeability. The "natural barriers" in the skin, which are formed by these fatty acids, appeared to be out of action and their ability to resist potential dangers was lowered.

EFA, used to treat some skin complaints, have produced remarkable results. In a letter to the *British Medical Journal,* Dr. C. Petit reported that he had used unsaturated fatty acids in treatment of psoriasis. One case healed completely in three months; after eighteen months the disease had not reappeared. Dr. Petit said he had also used unsaturated fatty acids in treatment of leg ulcers, with satisfactory results.

Having touched on the effects of EFA, positive and negative, on the skin, let us pass on to consider possible dangers to the nerves from EFA deficiency. The fatty sheath of the nerves is rich in unsaturated fatty acids, which means—of course—that it must have generous supplies in order to keep up to standard. In the absence, or insufficiency, of EFA, abnormal compounds might be formed in the system and the function of the nerves almost certainly would be disturbed in some way. Many doctors believe that there is a connection between EFA deficiency and diseases such as disseminated sclerosis. This latter is almost entirely a disease of "civilized" countries; it is practically unknown in India and in China. Mental diseases, which are rapidly increasing, are thought to have a similar cause.

And then, ulcers. Ulcers have been produced experimentally in animals by feeding them a diet lacking in EFA. Cases of duodenal ulcers are on the increase, *particularly in men.*

I mentioned earlier the medical belief that there is a relationship between diseases of the arteries and EFA. It used to be thought that the total fat in the diet must be considered in assessing the role of fat in arterial complaints. But now the general opinion seems to be that the operative factor is the amount eaten of "unnatural" fats (the hardened fats, including margarines, cooking fats, and shortenings), complicated by EFA deficiency.

However, I have noticed that a number of well-known Continental doctors, including the famous endocrinologist Professor Dreyfus, avoided cream with their meals, and merely scraped butter on bread. Apparently, they were playing safe.

We who mean to live out our full span also ought to play safe; perhaps not so drastically as these men, but we must watch the amount and type of fats in the diet. That doesn't mean that you have to say good-by forever to cream, if you are a man. You can let yourself go, and have a little now and again. But you would be well advised not to make a habit of cream-eating. In the strawberry season, I am particularly glad I am not a man.

None of us should overload the system with fat of any kind. But some fat the body must have, and that fat must contain unsaturated fatty acids. I have mentioned sources of EFA already; I would suggest that you should take wheat-germ oil every day, and halibut-liver oil. Also olive oil, or sunflower-seed oil on salads.

Beware of "hidden" fats which boost up your day's quota of fats toward the danger-line. "Hidden fats" are fats used in cooking, and are an ingredient of cakes, puddings, pastry, and foods of this sort. I would attach the largest-sized *beware* label to the frying-pan. That I always refer to as a lethal weapon. Its regular use is unjustifiable homicide. Frying destroys Vitamin F and the fat-soluble vitamins, such as A, E, and K. It increases the calorie value of food. As most people tend to have a high-calorie diet, this usually means an overstepping of the day's calorie quota. My slogan is "No calories without vitamins and minerals," which insures that fullest use is being made of calorie intake.

When fat is essential to a cooking process, use either olive oil, sunflower-seed oil, or lard, if possible. And don't forget the part played by whole-meal bread and flour in relation to EFA in the system. The whole-meal habit is an eating habit which one cannot afford not to acquire, if one is interested in living long and in good health.

Whole-meal bread contains the two vitamins particularly essential in connection with EFA in the system, as I have said. But one would have to eat uncomfortably large quantities of it in order to make sure of filling the day's complete requirements. It is simpler and safer, from this point of view, to take about three tablespoonsful of brewers' yeast every day. This is one of the best sources of all the B vitamins, among which is Vitamin B_6 (pyridoxine).

For extra Vitamin E (to ensure that you are getting sufficient of this vitamin daily), take wheat-germ oil or sunflower-seed oil. Vitamin E is not only a vital vitamin for utilization of EFA; the muscles need it, including the heart. In these days, more and more people seem to have heart trouble in one form or another. The regular use of Vitamin E, at least once the thirty mark is passed, is a commonsense health precaution. It can help to keep the heart young, in conjunction with Vitamin B, which the heart needs as well.

SUMMARY

FATS ARE NECESSARY TO NUTRITION, but intake of too much of the wrong kind or not enough of the right kind can seriously undermine your personal program for long life and long youth.

- learn the importance of the EFA—essential fatty acids
- consider any fats that do not contain Vitamin F "wrong"
- distrust and don't use "commercial" fats; stick with the cholesterol-free vegetable oils
- beware the frying pan

CHAPTER

7

MINERALS AND
LONG YOUTH

O N THIS PLANET, earth and air and water are built up
from ninety-two mineral elements. So, it would seem,
is the rest of the universe. Light rays from the stars, when
analyzed, have been found to contain these elements. And
we, our bodies, are made of the same stuff. We may be
dust—but dust with a difference; star dust.

No doubt all these minerals are necessary to whatever
processes are going on in other planets; certainly they are
necessary to the processes of our bodies. At one time, when
this or that mineral was discovered in our tissues not very
much notice was taken. The mineral was just "there"; its
presence was not recognized as being necessary to any particular function. Even now some textbooks talk about certain minerals as if they had got into the body by chance,

and as though there were no real reason why they should be present.

But the constantly advancing science of biochemistry has shown these elements as essential to the body's health. Many of them are present in such microscopic amounts that they are almost undetectable. The presence of some, in even smaller quantities, can only be deduced through the behavior of other elements, much as the presence of new planets was deduced before they were found.

Gallium and germanium are two of these rare metals. Both are related to the health of the blood; gallium is used in biochemic therapy when blood formation is faulty. Germanium has been found to act beneficially on the red blood corpuscles, and on the bone marrow. It is considered a blood cell nutrient.

These minerals are present in the soil. They reach us by a natural process of transference through plants, vegetables, fruit, and water; or, one degree farther removed from source, through the flesh of animals or birds—or through eggs.

Minerals, let me repeat, are vital to health. The soil ought to supply all our needs, and if it did, we would probably be much healthier than we are—or at least the opportunity for better health would be there.

But, for one reason or another, Mother Earth often lets us down. Deficiencies of some mineral in some place are often being discovered. The classic example is the iodine deficiency in Derbyshire, England, which was the underlying cause of the goiter, so general in that part of the country that it was called "Derbyshire neck." In some parts of Australia, the soil is cobalt-deficient, with the result that grazing cattle and sheep develop a form of anemia and die unless the lack is made good. There is a boron deficiency in some parts of Tasmania; the apple trees get a disease called "internal cork" if they are not given a preventive dose of borax. It works out at one pound per tree every four years. Not enough to make any difference? But it makes a difference to the apple trees. They keep free from "internal cork."

There is another reason why we cannot trust the soil to give us the minerals we need, even those of which we use minute quantities. The chemistry of the soil works on something like the same lines as that of the body; if the acid-alkaline balance is disturbed, a number of things go wrong. When the soil is too alkaline, plants and grass may not be able to take up trace elements even when these are present. Too much lime, for instance, can result in manganese starvation for vegetation. And then you find chlorosis, a sort of "plant anemia" (loss of green color), "speckled yellow" in sugar beets, "gray speck" in oats and wheat, and "marsh spot" in peas. Cattle and human beings eating these vegetables or cereals would be likely in their turn to suffer from manganese deficiency.

The most usual reason for over alkalinity of the soil is the use of artificial fertilizers and indiscriminate liming. Some form of control of this "terracide" is overdue. The policy of the British Soil Association, with which I am in wholehearted agreement, is to guard and cultivate by research and in every possible way the health and wellbeing of the soil. Lady Eve Balfour, Field Director of the Soil Association, says: ". . . plants can only reach their maximum vitality when grown in fully vitalized soil, and that soil can only reach its maximum vitality when it is fed with the waste products of fully vitalized plants and animals. For one thing is very certain: we cannot create vitality in a laboratory."

We cannot get away from the fact that the health and vitality of the soil is our own health, a point made by the Professor of Human Physiology at the University of Adelaide, Sir Cedric Stanton Hicks, M.Sc., Ph.D., M.D., F.R.I.C. He said: "It is everybody's business to realize that what the farmer grows will be in their bodies, and their bodies' health and strength, tomorrow."

But until the day dawns when scientists realize that they do not yet know enough to "improve," or even to reproduce the intricate chemistry of nature, we cannot depend upon the soil, as I have said, as a source of essential minerals. Or of vitamins, for that matter—but we will come to that point later on. For the moment, the answer seems to be to make use of the discoveries of biochemistry and to take mineral food supplements as a guard against shortages. Some minerals are of particular interest to us, because, although all of them are necessary to the achievement of a positive health standard, a few of them have been highlighted as being very, very valuable to long youth.

CALCIUM

Dr. Henry C. Sherman Mitchell, Professor Emeritus of Chemistry at Columbia University, is among the eminent scientists who believe that calcium is one of the most important minerals for long health and for long life. Hundreds of laboratory experiments have shown that a calcium-rich diet significantly increased the life span of rats. Sherman says that the laboratory rats are sufficiently similar in their nutritional chemistry to us "to throw light upon problems of human nutrition." Human beings show similar improvements in health and general conditions when their diets are supplemented along the same lines. As yet, of course, it has not been possible to determine if their life span will be increased beyond "normal" expectation, but to judge from their improved standard of health, it seems at least a possibility.

There are many other food factors to be considered in longevity; calcium is not the only mineral to contribute toward longer life. But it is, as I have said, a very important factor in health and nutrition, and can do much to help us to achieve our full life span. "Calcium deficiency," said one medical authority, "contributes to disease that precedes 90 per cent of all deaths."

J. T. Irving, M.A., Ph.D., F. Odont. Soc., S.A., Professor of Experimental Odontology, says: "Calcium is the most important inorganic element in the body, and occurs in the largest amount." Yet, according to Sherman, calcium deficiency is much more frequent than is generally thought. He says that on diets which appear to be reasonably adequate, but which do not contain liberal calcium, there may be every appearance of good health, even by the test of careful physical examination. In spite of this, because of the calcium shortage, sooner or later some form of ill health will develop. A surprising number of autopsies, he says, on people believed to be well nourished, reveal osteoporosis, a condition in which holes develop in the bones when calcium is lacking in the system and the body draws on its "banks," the bones and the teeth. The bones are a very rich supply of this mineral. They have a kind of delicate internal latticework of calcium, called trabec-

ulae, on which the system can draw for a supply of calcium when necessary. But there comes a time when the
"account" is overdrawn and calcium bankruptcy results.

You may be lacking in calcium because you are not eating enough of the foods which contain enough calcium.
Or you may not be absorbing it. Eating calcium is one
thing; getting the system to make use of it is another. You
might be swallowing quite a quantity of calcium, yet getting next to no good out of it because it is not being
assimilated.

One way or another, it is easy to go short of calcium.
Even a diet which apparently contains enough of this
mineral can let you down, if you don't watch points. For
one thing, calcium is lost in the kitchen. In cooking vegetables by the usual method of boiling, about 25 per cent
of the calcium content is leached away. This is not so serious if the water is kept and either drunk as it is, or used
in soups and gravy. But invaluable minerals—not only calcium and vitamins—too often are fed daily to the unap-
preciative sink. And that means a reduction in the day's
quota of dietary necessities. By the way, the outer—the
greenest—leaves of vegetables have most calcium in them.
It's a great waste to throw them away and eat only the
inner leaves, or heart, which contain less calcium than the
outer leaves. Among vegetables, collards, kale, turnip-tops,
and dry beans are the richest sources of this mineral.
Among nuts, almonds rate top place.

But to know which sources of calcium the body will
make use of and which it will not is even more important
than to know what percentage of the mineral is contained
in different foods. It obviously doesn't matter so much
from the point of view of nutrition if the calcium value

of a food is extremely high on paper; what does matter is how much of that calcium is what is called "available" to the system. An example is spinach, which—as I mentioned earlier—contains so much oxalic acid that, by combining with the calcium in the body, it can make the calcium useless nutritionally. The calcium in spinach is in the form of oxylate and is quite unavailable to the system. Sherman says of spinach: "Spinach is a mistaken choice for popularization as a typical green-leaf vegetable." Yet, as we all know, spinach is widely supposed to be particularly good for young children (who need every vestige of calcium they can get). It is even sold in specially prepared *purée* form for babies. Popeye the Sailor, the spinach addict, was toothless, you remember—which just shows what spinach can do for us.

Generally speaking, the full calcium content of vegetables is not available to the human body. About 13.4 per cent of the calcium content of carrots is used in the system. You would have to eat 700 grams of carrots to get a quarter of the day's quota. The calcium of lettuce is well utilized, but the content-value is not high; so again, you would have to get through an uncomfortably large amount of lettuce in order to reach the nutritional Plimsoll line. Incidentally, the method of growing vegetables influences their composition. Artificial fertilizers tend to lower the calcium element.

Milk and milk products (except butter) are the best sources of calcium, with vegetables and fruit as a necessary "make-weight." Goats' milk contains a little more of the mineral than does cows' milk. Cheese and milk (goats' or cows') are "musts" for a long-life diet plan.

Very well, then. We know that milk and cheese are our best means of getting enough calcium, because they contain reasonable amounts of the mineral in a form in which the body can make use of it. Now we have to make sure that the calcium will stay with us, so to speak. Certain conditions are favorable to calcium retention, others are not. You remember that a too-alkaline soil tended to prevent plants from taking up trace elements? A too-alkaline intestinal tract works in something like the same way, and reduces calcium absorption. Acidity—in reasonable, not excess amounts—in the digestive tract helps calcium absorption. For this reason, oranges are an aid to stacking up your calcium reserves. Oranges contain calcium themselves, but it is the action of the juice which is particularly valuable in this case. The juice is acid in the digestive tract; that takes care of the calcium. After the juice is dealt with, the acid salts are "burned" and reduced to an alkaline ash, which decreases the acidity of the body, thus helping to keep the acid-alkaline balance steady.

Cereals can be calcium-robbers. They contain a substance called phytic acid, which makes calcium insoluble and useless in the body. Oatmeal is the worst offender; it can decalcify the calcium content of the other foods in the diet. Cane sugars can interfere with calcium absorption, because they dissolve in the stomach and produce an alkaline condition. Chocolate and cocoa are "anticalcium." Avoid them.

Then there is the relation of Vitamin D to calcium. Its presence is absolutely essential to enable the system to make use of the mineral. It helps nullify the effects of the various anticalcifying substances that have been mentioned; it is a regulator of the vital calcium-phosphorus balance in the body.

Not many foods contain useful quantities of Vitamin D. The skin is able to manufacture it in the presence of certain light rays, but since in many parts of the world we rarely expose enough of our bodies to enough sunlight, the best thing to do is to take cod-liver oil or halibut-liver oil as a food supplement. Every day, as well as a fish-liver oil, take eggs, milk, and lettuce. Liver should appear on the menu as often as possible. By eating these foods, the effects of anticalcifying elements in your diet will be counteracted.

Before we go on, I would like to say, *à propos* eggs, that in order to have any value as Vitamin D containing foods, the hens which produce them must live in the open air, and be exposed to light. The bodies of hens cannot synthesize Vitamin D in the absence of natural light, any more than ours can. This is one reason why the system of keeping hens in batteries, indoors, should be ended. It is only one of many reasons—but I must not begin telling you about them now. We must get back to our minerals.

Calcium is necessary to many of the physical functions. It is an important mineral in the building and maintenance of bones and teeth; also for the functioning and development of other tissues. It regulates the heartbeat; the muscles cannot relax as they should without it, nor can the nerves. If you sleep badly, you may be calcium-deficient. Instead of taking sleeping pills or drugs of any kind if you are tense or highly strung, try the effect of calcium. It is easy to take, in tablet or in biochemic form. If taking the tablets, it is a good idea to swallow them with *fresh* orange juice—not in any preserved form. If taken with orange juice, it is a good plan to wash the mouth out afterward to prevent any possible damage to the teeth from undisturbed contact with the acid in the juice.

Calcium deficiency can produce muscular spasms or cramp, tetany, and some "rheumatic" pain in joints or muscles. Calcium is also indicated in cases of poor circulation, and it is beneficial in debility. It is particularly important in growing children; nervous, backward, and difficult children are often calcium-poor and improve amazingly when the deficiency is remedied. It has been found that girls are more likely to lack calcium than boys and need more of this mineral. In fact, an unstable calcium balance has been labeled as "characteristic of femininity."

PHOSPHORUS

Calcium and phosphorus are the Siamese twins in the mineral world. Like love and marriage, in the words of the song, "they go together like a horse and carriage," and "you can't have one without the other." Or, if you could, at any rate in the case of calcium and phosphorus, the results would be disastrous. Calcium and phosphorus are usually found together in foods, although meat is a good source of phosphorus, but not of calcium. We need about one and a half times as much phosphorus as calcium, and it is important to maintain an approximate balance; otherwise the body draws on its "bone-bank" to restore equilibrium. Fortunately Vitamin D, as I have said, regulates the balance of these minerals, keeping us out of the danger zone.

Phosphorus is important to the nerves, and for energy

production. In cases of TB it is valuable. *Also it is a factor in keeping the aging processes at bay.* Make a note of phosphorus, and be sure you get your full quota of this mineral daily. Its chief food sources are meat, as I have already mentioned, oysters, peanuts, peanut butter, radishes, salmon, sardines, brown rice, shrimps, soya beans, walnuts, wheat.

IRON

Iron is vital to the health of our blood; without iron we would not live very long. And yet it constitutes, at a maximum, only one ten-thousandth part of the human adult body—quantity does not mean a thing when assessing the value of minerals in the system. But although we need only such microscopic amounts of iron in our tissues, iron deficiency is very common. Anemia is a classic example of iron deficiency. Debility, lack of energy, pale lips and skin —and *aging*—are other signs of iron shortage. The mineral strengthens and rejuvenates the red corpuscles, and can be of benefit in cases of tuberculosis.

Iron is essential for hemoglobin formation, which gives the blood its red color, and which is composed of iron in combination with a protein. The red corpuscles are made in the marrow of bones; they enter the blood and circulate for about six weeks. Then they disintegrate, and their iron content passes to the liver, where it is stored until required. Iron is necessary to all cell functions.

We lose iron in sweat, in the feces, from cells sloughed from the skin, and from internal surfaces. None is lost in urine because the kidneys retain it.

The daily requirement is set at about 15 milligrams, but we should aim at getting at least twice that amount in our food. Most of us are likely to have too little iron than too much in our systems; we are borderline deficiency cases, and actual deficiency is widespread. The chief reason is that, like calcium, iron absorption is not easy for the body. In its organic form, the body cannot make use of iron. The iron in most meat is organic, so is over three-quarters of the iron content of cereals. In white fish, iron is inorganic, and so can be taken up by the body; the best sources are green vegetables, turnip-tops, mustard and cress, liver, kidney, eggs, watercress, dandelion leaves, shellfish, currants, raspberries, loganberries, yellowstone fruit, all dried fruits, and black molasses.

Iron, like calcium, is made unavailable to the system by oxalic acid and phytic acid, which is another reason why we should budget for at least twice the officially adequate amount of iron in our diet. It is not likely that we shall get the full iron ration contained in any item of food, even when it is in digestible form. Some of it will be put out of action by these two acids; also the sources of iron may not contain as much as they should, because the soil may be poor in iron. As with calcium, plants cannot take up iron if the soil is too alkaline or if it is short of humus. Sometimes plants and fruit have been found to have only one-sixth of the amount of iron which they should contain. I repeat that in order to make sure of getting 15 milligrams of iron in our food, we may have to eat two or three times that amount. Even when we have achieved our iron quota, copper and Vitamin C are both necessary to its full utilization in the system.

COBALT

The discovery of the importance of cobalt in nutrition is comparatively recent. Cobalt is a constituent of Vitamin B_{12}, which has been used with great success in treatment of certain forms of anemia. When cobalt is deficient in soil, as it is in certain parts of Australia, animals there develop a wasting disease, from which they die. If cobalt is given, they recover. Cobalt, as we know, is essential to the healthy functioning of the pancreas, as well as the red blood corpuscles.

ZINC

Zinc is an important factor in the processes of digestion; again a comparatively recent discovery. The blood and muscles contain it; muscular control requires its presence, both in the muscles and in the brain. Dr. Henry Gilbert, the eminent biochemist, says that "zinc seems to stimulate the chemical mechanism by which the body maintains its acid-base equilibrium, and also helps the blood to deal with a number of diseases."

Zinc is a constituent of insulin, which is essential to the process of sugar utilization in the body. We need 10 to 15 milligrams daily. The best food sources are wheat germ and wheat-bran. If we eat white bread, we run the risk of zinc shortage. *Zinc is a "must" for long life.*

BORON

This mineral is present in our bodies in minute quantities. In plants, its function is concerned with the circulatory health. Its work in the human body is considered to be similar, but this is not completely established. Generally speaking, we are not likely to be boron-deficient. As we get older, our bodies retain it in greater quantities.

ALUMINUM

This is the third most important mineral in the composition of the soil, but in living tissue, it is one of the scarcest; about one part in a million is the figure. Mosses and ferns seem to be aluminum addicts. They are the only plants which take it up in large quantities. Since we do not eat ferns or land mosses, we can write them off as danger sources of excess aluminum. But from aluminum saucepans, jelly-molds, or other cooking utensils a relatively large quantity of aluminum can pass into the body. Within the past few years a crusade has come into being against the use of this type of kitchen ware. The best plan, I would say, is to play safe. Use aluminum pots and pans as little as possible, but do not worry if temporarily you can't avoid them—for instance, if you happen to stay with people who won't listen to a word against them. The reason is that you can almost say that the body rejects aluminum. Neither calcium nor iron is absorbed easily by the body, but compared with its absorption of aluminum it soaks up these minerals.

COPPER

This mineral is particularly vital to health. Iron must have copper if it is to work efficiently in the body. Unless copper is present, the iron stored in the liver cannot be converted into hemoglobin. Animal liver is a good source of the metal, so are nuts. Research has shown that dark hair has more copper in it than light-colored hair. And also that if the copper level decreases, hair loses pigment and turns gray.

ARSENIC

In the course of about a month or six weeks we take a fatal dose of arsenic into our systems. Both men and soil contain arsenic, and it is found in all plant and animal tissue. White sugar is supposed to be the only food which is without it. In the amounts in which it normally is present in our systems it is essential. It prevents waste and loss of phosphorus and corrects faulty phosphorus metabolism. Some authorities believe that many cases of allergy may be explained by arsenic deficiency.

FLUORINE

This mineral salt is necessary for the brain, the bones, and the teeth, but an excess can cause havoc. Bones and teeth can be seriously affected by too much fluorine; spinal trouble can be another result. Fluorine is the most chemically active of the elements. It is present in drinking water and in plant and animal tissues.

SULPHUR

Sulphur occurs in protein in amounts sufficient to make it likely that anyone whose diet is about average will get enough sulphur for the body's needs. Sulphur is antiseptic and purifying. It spreads to all parts of the body as sulphurous gas. It is valuable in skin diseases, intestinal infections, bronchial diseases, rheumatism, and infection of the pilary gland (alopoecia).

VANADIUM

This substance is necessary to the blood in very small quantities. It stimulates and increases the action of the phagocytes, the cells which guard the body against infection. And biochemistry has discovered that, in conjunction with other minerals, *it works to prevent aging.*

SODIUM AND POTASSIUM

These are very closely related, and the sodium-potassium balance is of great importance to the health of all the cells. More sodium than potassium is necessary to the body, but excess of either element could be disastrous. We all need salt; it is a constituent of our blood, which tells the story of our ancestry. We came out of the sea originally; it is with us still, in our arteries and in our veins. The chemical constitution of our blood is similar to that of the oceans in which, millions of years ago, the life of this planet began. The percentage of the elements in our blood approximates that of the ancient seas; it contains far less magnesium than is found in the oceans today; their magnesium content has increased since our earliest ancestors left in search of better living accommodation. The primeval formula survives in our blood streams.

The average person's sodium requirement is assessed at

4 grams daily. Most people add about four times that amount to their food, at table. That is in addition to what the cook has put in. The moral of this is—try to forget the salt-cellar at meals. It is risky to overload the system with sodium; the safest plan is to change from ordinary table salt to a compound of mineral salts, scientifically balanced to correspond to the chemical balance of the body.

Potassium is essential to the healthy functioning of all muscles; especially the heart. It stimulates the nerves and alkalinizes overacidity of the stomach and blood. It is a factor in generating cellular electricity and it is anticonstipation. It is widely distributed in plant and animal tissue, so that a normal mixed diet is not likely to be short of it.

IODINE

The minimum daily amount necessary to health of this mineral is 75 milligrams. It is found in seafood (ocean fish), and in sea-greens, also in watercress, lettuce, onion, leeks, artichokes, and melon. To make sure of getting your daily ration of this important mineral salt, which helps to keep you youthfully vigorous and on top of the world, take some form of Irish moss dried carrageen daily. This moss is sold dried, or in flake form. It may be added to soups and stews; it can be used for thickening sauces, making blanc-manges, and jellies. It is a most useful and valuable addition to the diet. Children and adolescents need more iodine than adults, but iodized sweets are not a safe way of increasing their ration. Children are apt to eat too many, which could result in iodine intoxication.

Iodine, as we have seen earlier, is essential to the thyroid

gland. It also relieves congestion and helps in the formation of the "guardian cells," the phagocytes.

SILICA

The blood must contain approximately ten parts per
million of silica. When this percentage sinks, you begin to
feel "under the weather"; you probably get cold feet, in
every sense, because the morale sinks with the body temperature. The hair becomes thin and brittle; baldness may
be due to it, and lack of body heat may be entirely caused
in this way. The skin loses its elasticity; silica is a constituent of the connective tissue, including the supportive
tissue of the lungs. We have already mentioned the vital
importance of the connective tissue to the prolongation of
youth, health, and life, so silica is of particular interest as
an aid to reaching our 180th birthdays.

Silica, which is a dioxide of the element silicon, is a
colorless substance, and it is more abundant than any
other solid element of our globe. Flint, sandstone, rock
crystal, quartz, and chalcedony are examples of silica. The
opal belongs to the same family. The action of sun and
rain and frost through millions of ages has ground down
silica substances into minute particles in the soil. Silica is
the supportive element which gives to wheat strength to
stand upright. For both strength and normality of form,
silica is necessary to plants—and to us.

Silica is present in most parts of our bodies. But, as we
grow older, the amount of this element in the system decreases, the only biological element to behave in this way.
Carbonates are substituted for silica, a chemical change of
age. In young people, the skin has been found to contain

50 milligrams per kilogram; in old people it decreases to 40 per kilogram.

The brittleness of bones in the elderly is not only due to calcium deficiency; lack of silica can be the cause. When fingernails are weak and thin, silica as well as calcium should be supplied. Teeth also need it; so do the muscles and the eyes. The lens of the eye contains twenty-five times as much silica as do the muscles, and homeopaths claim that there is a type of cataract which is cured by silica. In the days of Paracelsus, silica was used as a remedy for asthma, lung troubles, and coughs.

Silica has been used in the treatment of cancer and of sarcoma. Dr. H. H. Patrick of Glasgow has reported cases of sarcoma cured by silica. Dr. George Burford says that ". . . the leading features of the healing process [of malignant growths] is the reaction of the connective tissue. It is by speeding up the antagonistic powers of connective tissue [by silica] that the natural cures of malignancy, partial or entire, are largely effected."

Malnutrition, epilepsy, rheumatism, obesity, and arteriosclerosis are other complaints in the treatment of which silica has produced good results.

I do not believe that one single mineral, one vitamin, one anything, can be a complete answer to our quest. But silica can make a contribution of such value that it should have a prominent place in our present plan. Fortunately silica, unlike iron and calcium, is easily absorbed. The body will take it up, even in old age, which is a vital point. It occurs in the skin of fruit, in the outer shell of cereals, and the skin of potatoes. Nearly all vegetables have some quantity of it; it is usually to be found in or near the skin, which is another reason for not peeling fruit or vegetables unless it is unavoidable. Asparagus, artichokes, celery, cucumber, dandelion, leeks, milk, oats, radishes, sunflower seeds, tomatoes, and turnips are all good sources of silica. And among herbs, field horsetail (*equisetum arvense*) is in a class by itself. Houndtongue (*cyneglossum officinale*), lungwort (*pulmonaria officinale*), comfrey (*symphytus officinale*), and herbnettle (*galeopsis orchrileuca*) are excellent sources of the mineral. You should be able to get a supply of these herbs at any herbalist's shop and at most health stores.

If you gather the herbs yourself, the best plan is to lay in as large a stock as possible of them all, or as many as you can find. Dry the leaves over the cooking stove, spread on paper, or in an airing cupboard. Then pack them into glass jars with tightly fitting lids. Make "tea" with these dried leaves by pouring boiling water over about an egg-cupful of herbs (mixed). It is best to let the brew stand until cold, then drink it. Two or three cupfuls should be taken daily. You do not need to bother about the exact proportion of comfrey, lungwort, and other herbs in each brew. They mix quite happily.

There are any number of other minerals—nickel, nitre, chromium, and manganese among them—which occur in minute but vital amounts in our bodies. They are found in plant and animal tissues, and it is unlikely that there would be any shortage of them in our diet.

I am sure you realize how important it is to long life and long youth that there should be no shortage of any mineral in our food. Make sure of your daily ration, and watch your energy, vitality, and general wellbeing improve, together with your chances of scoring 180 birthdays.

SUMMARY

MINERALS ARE PART of the intricate and fascinating chemistry of life. Like vitamins, minerals are vital to our program. Of some we have easily an adequate intake in a balanced diet; others we need to supplement. With some minerals, as with some vitamins, the problem is not only of getting what we need but also of making certain we retain and assimilate what we need.

The chief food sources of the minerals discussed in this chapter will be found listed in the Appendix.

Sixteen minerals of importance to good and long life are
- calcium
- phosphorus
- iron
- cobalt
- zinc
- boron
- aluminum
- copper
- arsenic
- fluorine
- sulphur
- vanadium
- sodium
- potassium
- iodine
- silica

CHAPTER

8

THE MAGIC OF VITAMINS

Magic, says the *Oxford Dictionary*, is an "inexplicable or remarkable influence, producing surprising results." That is just what vitamins could be said to be—and do. Since the more or less "official" discovery of the anti-neuritic vitamin (shortened to "aneurin") B_1 by Dr. Casimir Funk in 1912, vitamins have established themselves as remarkable (and in many cases, still not fully explained) influences, producing surprising results in human health. All the vitamins are found in foodstuffs, so that, even although they can be produced synthetically, they belong primarily to the "new" science of nutrition rather than to medicine. But they are now used so widely in the treatment of so many different diseases that they have breeched the artificial division that has been built up between the two sciences of eating and healing. In the days of Hippocrates and Galen there was no such divorce between them; these great physicians realized the vital relationship which exists between food and health. "Let your medicine be your food and your food your medicine," said Galen.

Everybody nowadays knows about vitamins. They have helped to make us food-conscious in a useful way; that is, to realize that the right food, not just any food, is necessary to keep us healthy. No discovery is valuable unless it is accepted and made use of; the news value of vitamins has been of good service to nutrition in this way.

Vitamins could be described as the sparks which set bodily processes going and enable them to keep going. Vitamins are essential to health, and life, and youth. Nutrition scientists tell us that what we think of as aging can be a premature process, due to a lack in our diet of essentials—which include vitamins. They claim that, by adequate supply in diet of these essentials, aging processes can be retarded and reversed.

Dr. Tom Spies, to whom I have already referred, one of the greatest names in nutritional research, who has the Gold Medal of the American Medical Association, plus a citation (the Distinguished Service Award), said at the 1957 convention of the American Medical Association: "If only we knew enough, all diseases could be prevented, and could be cured, through proper nutrition." Of the process of aging, his opinion is: "As tissues become damaged because they lack the chemicals [vitamins and such] of good nutrition, they tend to become old. They lack what I call 'tissue integrity.' . . . If we can help the tissues repair themselves by correcting nutritional deficiencies, we *can make old age wait.*" (Italics mine).

Dr. Spies' method of treating patients by diet and diet

supplements only produced wonderful results. I have already referred to this "mass cure" of the 873 people in Birmingham, Alabama, who were brought to his nutrition clinic after they had been given up by their own doctors as hopeless cases.

As with minerals, so among vitamins some are classed as star performers as regards "making old age wait," and helping generally to prolong the life span. But although these particular vitamins may be cast for the leading role in some ways, let me say once more that every vitamin, every mineral and every element of diet—protein, starches, sugars, fats—is vital to keeping young and healthy—and alive.

Here is a brief ABC of vitamins and their properties.

RIBOFLAVIN

I am putting this vitamin first because Professor Sherman considers that it is a major factor in prolonging life and the prime of life. "Riboflavin deficiency [*ariboflavinosis*]," he says, "is one of the most common deficiencies in many countries." Unlike a shortage of its fellow vitamin and co-worker Vitamin B_1 (thiamine or aneurin) riboflavin deficiency takes a long time to show up. Symptoms of its shortage in a child (it is essential to growth) might be written off as "backwardness," inherent inability to develop at a normal rate, and similar symptoms. McLeod and Taylor say that the end result of deficiency would be a shortening of life and premature senility.

Riboflavin is the "skin" vitamin. It is an important factor in keeping the skin smooth and healthy, and since the origin of the eye is a specially developed skin spot, it is essential to the eyes, as one might expect. It can have amazing results in the treatment of sore, inflamed eyes, eyes which water in cold winds, and similar conditions. In such cases, it is a good plan to take 3 milligrams of riboflavin before each meal.

Even though you may think you are eating plenty of riboflavin-containing foods, you may not be getting your quota, perhaps because the foods themselves may be short of their riboflavin content. This vitamin is sensitive to light; for instance, milk stored in plain glass bottles in daylight loses quite a percentage of its riboflavin. Amber coloring should be the rule for milkbottles—but that is another story. As I was saying, you may be deficient in riboflavin for one reason or another; sometimes even if the diet is in theory and in fact up to standard as regards this vitamin, the body's chemistry may not be functioning on all cylinders, so to speak, and you may not be absorbing riboflavin properly. A doctor who took great care to eat correctly still suffered from inflamed eyes. The trouble cleared up completely after a course of riboflavin. In my own case, a sty (the only one I've ever had) gave me a couple of days of discomfort, until I realized that I might need extra riboflavin. A few hours after taking the vitamin, the sty decreased till it was hardly visible. Within twenty-four hours it had disappeared.

Deficiency of riboflavin causes digestive disturbances and nervous troubles, general weakness, debility, and lack of energy. Resistance to disease is lowered. If it persists, the life span is likely to be shortened.

The right amount of riboflavin in the diet builds you up. It gives energy and vitality, helps digestion and nerves to function well, strengthens the eyes, and affords resistance to disease. Finally, its action is in the direction of prolonging life and the prime of life.

Broccoli, cabbage, kale, fresh peas, apples, almonds, green beans, potatoes, tomatoes, turnips, wheat, liver, beef, eggs, milk, cheese, are good sources of this vitamin, especially the last five items.

THIAMINE (B₁)

Vitamin B_1 is, as I pointed out earlier, particularly essential as co-worker with riboflavin. In fact, all the B vitamins are so closely connected that they must be considered as a group; to take one of them alone increases the need for the others. So, when there is a marked deficiency of one or another of the group, the best way of dealing with it is to take yeast, which is a rich source of all the B vitamins, and then to take, in addition, the special B vitamin of which a shortage is indicated.

Vitamin B_1, or thiamine, is also known as aneurin, a portmanteau word made from a description of its first-discovered function; ANti-NEURitic-vitamIN. As its name implies, it is necessary to the health of the nervous system, and when it is deficient some form of nervous disorder is likely to appear. Whole wheat, and whole-meal bread and flour are the best sources; barley, oats, and beans come next. Asparagus is the vegetable which has most thiamine in it.

"Nerves," in some form or another, are today a general complaint. So are constipation and indigestion; these disorders can be symptoms of shortage of B_1. If you want to avoid them, get the habit of eating whole-meal instead of white bread, whole-meal flour, and whole-grain cereals. These thiamine-containing foods also help to keep your heart strong and active all your life; the heart must have thiamine.

Thiamine is sensitive to heat; cooking reduces its effectiveness. Contact with alkalines, such as bicarbonate of soda, destroys it.

PYRIDOXINE (B₆)

Pyridoxine is vital to our long-life plan for many reasons, of which a most important one is the part it plays in the utilization of unsaturated fatty acids in the system, as we have already seen. It, like thiamine, is found in whole-grain cereals, flour, and bread. Muscles need it, with calcium, in order to be able to function properly and to relax efficiently. If you find yourself tense, remember pyridoxine as well as calcium. It has also been discovered that pyridoxine deficiency can result in a dermatitis of the ear and in lowered resistance of the middle ear to infection. Dr. T. S. Gardner found that addition of pyridoxine to the diet of laboratory animals *increased their life span*.

PANTOTHENIC ACID

When pantothenic acid (another of the B group) was added to pyridoxine, the increased longevity in these animals was more marked. These two vitamins, plus yeast nucleic acid, brought the figure up to 46.6 per cent, or about half again as long as the accepted period of life.

FOLIC ACID AND B$_{12}$

Two of the B group, folic acid and Vitamin B$_{12}$ (erithrotin) are particularly necessary for blood health. Folic acid, with other members of the B group, helps to keep the hair from turning gray; B$_{12}$ is a wonderful "toner-up" of the system.

OTHER B GROUP MEMBERS

Inositol, choline, betaine, nicotinic acid (niacin), and para-aminobenzoic acid, all belong to this vitamin family and all play their part in the body's chemistry, enabling it to keep the vital processes going and to delay aging. All the B vitamins are musts in the long-life program.

The best way to put them on your diet is to include Vitamin B-rich foods on your menu every day. Yeast I have already mentioned; three to four tablespoonsful of dried brewers' yeast should be taken daily, either in soup, tomato juice, or in some other liquid. Yoghurt is another fine source of these vitamins and also of calcium. In Bulgaria, where long life is taken as a matter of course, yoghurt is looked upon as one of the prerequisites if you want to top the century mark. Black molasses is full of B vitamins and valuable minerals; so is wheat germ, which also has in it Vitamin E. Dried milk is rich in riboflavin; use it to increase the value of fresh milk, soups, and gravies. Sherman suggests that two quarts of milk is the optimal daily milk allowance for adults. While this would be desirable from the point of view of health, probably few of us could manage to drink so much milk daily. This is where powdered milk becomes useful. About half a cupful of dried milk equals the value of a quart of fresh milk. By combining fresh and dried milk, you can manage your two quarts without difficulty. But I must say again that dried milk is *not* a substitute for, and must be used *as well as,* not instead of, fresh milk. Being fat-free, dried skimmed milk adds its valuable quota to fresh milk without stepping up fat calories or cholesterol in the diet—another great advantage.

VITAMIN A

Vitamin A is one of the keep-young vitamins. It has been found that even in diets which contained "enough of everything," the addition of Vitamin A produced a higher health standard and longer life span in laboratory animals. "We need have no doubt," says Sherman, "that the same thing may often occur with people. . . . There is no doubt of [Vitamin A's] relation to health and longevity."

Vitamin A works in many important ways to keep us young. It is the main factor in the health of the cells which line our digestive, respiratory, and excretory tracts, and also the nose and lungs; and those which cover the eyes and the skin. All glands are covered with these cells, the epithelial cells. When Vitamin A is short in our bodies, deteriorations of the skin appear; colds, bronchial pneumonia, infectious illnesses, and glandular disorders such as kidney stone can result.

Eyes must have Vitamin A, not only for remedy against and prevention of night-blindness (for which it was used in the last war) but for their general health. The small raised spots which sometimes appear in the cornea of the eye (Bitot's spots) can be a symptom of Vitamin A deficiency and usually clear up when a sufficiency of the vitamin is taken.

Ears must have Vitamin A. Shortage can lead to ear infection and affect the mechanism of hearing. It is essential to the health of the kidneys and of the urinary tract to have adequate amounts of Vitamin A daily; this vitamin has been used with great effect in allergy therapy. It has been found that attacks of hay fever can generally be warded off by taking 150,000 units of Vitamin A before the attack develops. Allergies, by the way, as a rule only show themselves when the health is below par.

Mellanby reports from hospital experience that increased intake of Vitamin A decreases danger of infection; other doctors have called it the "first line of defense against illness" when taken in amounts about three to four times as much as was ordinarily thought adequate.

According to Kruse, deficiency of Vitamin A is much more common than was supposed until recently. Only within the last year or two has it been realized that Vitamin A shortage can make you "accident prone" by slowing up your reactions and attentiveness. Controlled tests were carried out in Karlsruhe, Germany, with 152 drivers who either could not pass their driving tests or who had an abnormally high accident record. These drivers were given 150,000 units of Vitamin A daily—which resulted, according to the Institute of Traffic Psychology in Karlsruhe, in "striking improvement in their driving proficiency." Control groups who were given placebos showed no change.

So, for quick response and alertness, general well being, and "long health," be liberal with Vitamin A.

Milk, butter, cream, cream cheeses, liver and kidneys,

are the best sources of Vitamin A. Green vegetables, some root vegetables and fruit contain carotene. This is called the "precursor" of Vitamin A—a substance which the system converts into the vitamin so that it can be absorbed by the body. When we assess the Vitamin A value of vegetables or fruit, we have to remember that only about one-third of their carotene content will become Vitamin A in the body, because our physical mechanism does not convert carotene easily. So that although on paper kale, broccoli and turnip greens are large shareholders in carotene, the amount of Vitamin A value resulting in the body will not be anything approaching the carotene content figure. The green outer leaves of vegetables—the leaves most people throw away—are the most valuable, as regards carotene supply. The greener the leaf, the more carotene and minerals it will contain. The heart of a lettuce has been found to have less than one-thirtieth the amount of Vitamin A (or carotene) contained in the outer, green leaves. The same is true of cabbages and other vegetables.

VITAMIN C

Never go short of this vitamin. Apart from its importance to the general health, it is a vital factor as regards longevity—and long youth. It is essential to the formation and health of the intercellular tissues—the connective tissues, in other words. You remember that Alexander and Victor Bogomoletz and Professor Filatov, the great Russian biologists and gerontologists, believe that the connective tissue is the key to health and rejuvenation.

Therefore, abundant supplies of Vitamin C are important to our program. Vitamin C alone won't rejuvenate you, but it will help to provide what nutritionists call "the right internal environment." This vitamin has many important functions, besides its ability, as McCallum and Simmonds put it, of "conservation of the characteristics of youth." With Vitamin A, it is *the* great defense against infection. It inactivates toxins in the blood. Colds and coughs yield to it; if it is taken in large enough doses, it usually acts as a safeguard from these complaints and from flu, if the general health standard is reasonably good. But in order to get these results, you must use the "saturation" technique. In emergencies 50 milligrams every half-hour for twenty-four hours is the safest way of insuring that an effective amount of Vitamin C is available to the system. The Vitamin C level varies, even in normal health, from person to person, often from day to day. The presence of bacteria in the body lowers the Vitamin C level in the system. About 25 milligrams of the vitamin are used up when you smoke a cigarette. An outsize dose takes care of all these variables and possibilities, and insures that there is some over for use in other essential purposes. But the dose must be taken regularly; the system cannot store Vitamin C.

The muscles, teeth and gums, the sex organs, and glandular tissues need Vitamin C. It is necessary to calcium retention, to the blood, the bones, and the heart. It helps wounds to heal and aids resistance to physical stress.

The more protein you eat, the more Vitamin C you need. As I said a couple of paragraphs back, smoking increases the need of the system for the vitamin—a point which the Toronto nutritionist, Dr. McCormick, stresses.

Citrus fruits and green vegetables—watercress, cabbage, broccoli, turnip-tops—are all good sources of Vitamin C.

So are tomatoes, cantaloup melon, black currants, and rose-hips. Rose-hip tablets are an excellent way of providing a basic Vitamin C ration; they are on sale at many drugstores and most health stores. Make sure before buying them that the Vitamin C content per tablet is stated; otherwise you will not know how many tablets to take. It is better to take a natural product, if you can—such as rose-hips—always provided that white sugar is not used in its preparation. The alternative is ascorbic acid tablets, which any druggist stocks. Do not look on these tablets as anything but supplements; they are used as well as, not instead of, a diet rich in Vitamin C-containing foods. Every single day, you need at a minimum 400 milligrams of this vitamin; every single day, because, as I have said, Vitamin C cannot be stored in the body. You need not be afraid of taking an overdose; Vitamin C is nontoxic, however much is taken. The body simply excretes any of the vitamin which is in excess of its daily needs.

VITAMIN E

Vitamin E is usually known as the "fertility vitamin." There is no doubt that it is necessary to reproduction, but it is just as necessary to healthy functioning of the muscles and to the health of the heart, which is the most important muscle of all. Vitamin E has been used in the treatment of diabetes, and, recently, of asthma. Vitamin E is an antithrombin—it prevents or retards coagulation of the blood and so helps to keep veins and arteries clear of bloodclots. It strengthens capillaries so that hemorrhages are less likely, and it can dilate the veins. Two Canadian doctors, Stephen Tolgyes and Evan Shute, tell us in the

Canadian Medical Association's journal that where there is an obstruction of the circulation Vitamin E can produce a new blood vessel around the site of the obstruction, so that the blood can continue to circulate.

Vitamin E is a "must" for long life. Its best sources are wheat germ and wheat-germ oil, sunflower-seed oil, brown rice, eggs, and salads, especially lettuce, in which Vitamin E is found in conjunction with Vitamin A. These vitamins (A and E) work together, and one of them should not be taken without the other. Vitamin E is nontoxic, but if taken in massive doses it could increase the blood pressure in anyone suffering from that complaint who was not used to Vitamin E. A little should be taken to begin with, gradually working up to the required amount. As the vitamin is found only in small quantities in most foods, there is very little fear that our ordinary meals would boost Vitamin E intake to the danger mark.

VITAMIN D

Vitamin D's chief function is to promote absorption of calcium in the system and to regulate the balance between that mineral and phosphorus. It enables full utilization of both calcium and phosphorus by the body. It influences all the functions in which calcium and phosphorus are necessary. One of the most important is the body's ability to burn sugar, which cannot be achieved without phosphorus. For clotting of the blood, healthy heart action, and nervous stability Vitamin D is needed. Some eye diseases and some cases of arthritis have shown great improvement after treatment with Vitamin D. It is now thought that the healthy functioning of the thyroid gland is related to Vitamin D. Vitamin D deficiency increases the rate at which food is burned up, and since this is regulated by the thyroid gland, the amount of Vitamin D present in the system must affect the thyroid.

Bones and teeth are the special field of influence of Vitamin D, and so is the good posture that comes from good bones.

It is very difficult to get enough Vitamin D from diet; few foods contain any of this vitamin, and even when they do the content is low. Eggs, milk, butter, liver, herring and mackerel, salmon and tuna fish all have some Vitamin D, but the best source is fish-liver oil. Cod-liver oil is highest in Vitamin D, but contains less Vitamin A than halibut-liver oil. The latter oil is the better choice, because we need more Vitamin A than D. Halibut-liver oil should supply enough of both vitamins and should be taken the year round, except when—and if—you are able to be out of doors in the summer sunshine for two or three hours daily.

Vitamin D is the "sun" vitamin. There is a substance in our skin on which the ultraviolet rays act to produce Vitamin D. Then it is absorbed by the skin and circulates in the blood stream.

As soon as you get tanned, that is the end of your Vitamin D manufacture for that season—unless you get "untanned." Tan is nature's protection against an excess of ultraviolet light, so although a good tan looks healthy, in fact it is nothing of the sort. You will get the best value from sunshine if you stay as much as possible in the shade on a bright day.

Window-glass filters out the ultraviolet rays; clothing shuts them out from the skin. But you do not need to expose the whole surface of your body to sunlight, unless you want to. Vitamin D is manufactured in any part of the skin which the ultraviolet rays can reach and will then be carried by the blood to all parts of the body.

SPECIAL NOTE: If you are fair-skinned, you can get your Vitamin D ration in about half the time a dark-skinned type will need for production of the same amount of the vitamin.

If you want to make the most of Vitamin D, wash your hands as seldom as possible, and use the minimum of soap. Soap removes the oily secretions of the skin, and anything which removes these secretions also removes Vitamin D. Obviously we cannot go about dirt-encrusted—and that, in any case, would prevent Vitamin D formation—but we can cut down hand-washing as much as possible without breaking the laws of hygiene. Most people wash their hands far too often.

As regards the daily morning—or evening—bath, use as little soap as you can. It is not necessary to soap the whole body every day; total immersion (water-bath), and hand friction is enough. Friction with the hands does not remove the oils of the skin, it helps to stimulate their production, and to promote skin health—and youth and beauty.

SUMMARY

VITAMINS CAN BE CALLED the sparks that set bodily processes going and enable them to keep going. This chapter has been a brief *ABC* of vitamins and their properties. The chief food sources of vitamins can be found in the Appendix.

It would be oversimplifying to attempt to summarize by a single tag what each vitamin *does* primarily in human nutrition. You would be wiser to reread this chapter than try to remember one key function for each vitamin. For a quick reminder, however, here are the chief vitamins, as outlined in this chapter:

- Vitamin A
- The Vitamin B group
    Riboflavin
    Thiamine (B_1); also known as aneurin
    Pyridoxine (B_6)
    Pantothenic acid
    Folic acid
    B_{12} (Erithrotin)
- Vitamin C
- Vitamin D
- Vitamin E
- Vitamin F (see Chapter 6)

CHAPTER

9

RECIPE FOR REJUVENATION

ONE of the most spectacular ways of rejuvenating the appearance of the body is by the correct use of the muscles. The muscles are all ready for use. They can be put to work without elaborate preparations, merely by the influence of the mind, and when properly organized, they can perform seeming miracles.

They can reshape the body; they can lift sagging cheeks, melt away double chins, middle-aged spread "spare tires," and abdominal bulges. They restore elasticity to the skin, and make it smooth and healthy. They "iron out" crêpey necks. They dispose of flabbiness.

Flabbiness is a sign of weak, wasted muscles. And wasted muscles, says Dr. Edward Börtz, can cause premature old age. Dr. Börtz, who has been mentioned earlier in this book, is a former president of the American Medical Association; sixty-one himself, he believes that the average human life span should be a minimum of 150.

The right use of the muscles is one of the great secrets of youth—and health. The muscles have an enormously important job; they are the principal weight-carriers of the body; they support the vital organs. Poor or failing eye-sight can be due to slackening of the muscles of the face and eyes, in particular to those surrounding the eyes. The "set" of the eye in its socket can be affected by muscular deterioration. Strain results as the eye struggles to accommodate itself.

When we are young, if we are in normal health, we have a natural urge to use our muscles. We want to play games, dance, walk, and run. As we get into the thirties the pace slows. And not only are most of us less energetic, but also we use our muscles less energetically for those movements we do make. When we walk, we tend just to make enough effort to get along; we do not, generally speaking, use our legs from hip to toe, as they were made to be used, so that all the muscles are brought into play. As a result, the muscles weaken. Then fat forms—flabby fat.

This is the sort of thing that goes on in every part of the body. Muscles are only too ready to take the line of least resistance and do as little work as they can. Often the fore-arms—especially those of women—get flabby during the forties. In most cases, that is because when using the arms all the muscles are not being brought into play. Enough push and pull is not being put into even the movements which are made.

It does not help matters either, to use hands and arms for work for which they were not intended. Every day I

watch people hauling themselves up from chairs and bus
seats by hands and arms—a job which properly belongs
to the muscles of the diaphragm, abdomen, and thighs.
The muscles of the diaphragm in particular are enormously powerful, or should be. They should not need help
from hands or arms in raising the body from the sitting
position. But the less these muscles are used, the less
willing they are to be used, and eventually there comes
a time when they are so weak that it is hard manual labor
to get out of a chair.

This "helping hand" habit is insidious; very easy to get
into without noticing what is happening. Before you know
where you are, the hands are getting *SOS* messages from
muscles in other parts of the body, from the midriff, legs,
and thighs, to help them, for instance, lower the body into
a bath (they can legitimately ask for a little help in getting out of it); to raise you from a kneeling position, lift
you out of bed, and help you into it. And so it goes.

What we have to aim at—and not only aim at, but
achieve—if we want to make and keep ourselves supple
and youthful, is control of our muscles. That is what I
referred to at the beginning of this chapter as proper
organization. Once that has been done, we have a dynamic
force at our command.

This force will, literally, resurrect the body; resurrect it
in the dictionary sense of causing "revival from disuse, or
inactivity, or decay."

This method of organizing the muscles so that they
will obey us is based on a system of muscle control taught
by the Greeks in about the fifth century B.C. In those days,
the Greek race reached a peak of physical perfection which
was a byword; even today their beauty is legendary.

These early Greeks knew the importance of the muscular system to bodily health and symmetry. At the age of five, the Greek child began its training at the *palaestra* (the gymnasium). The child was taught not muscle development in the usual sense but the use of muscles. The result aimed at was a muscular condition which achieved perfect coordination and control. This made for a mastery of the body and its movements that few of us today would believe possible. The establishment of correct relationship between muscle and muscle, and their right use, meant that fatigue was almost abolished; what we should rate as feats of endurance could be carried out without strain.

The secret of achieving this state of coordination of the muscles is to establish a condition of tension.

Tension in this sense does not mean strain or stress or tenseness. Tension here is used in the sense in which it is used in mechanics, to mean the pull which is exercised by and on objects when they are part of a system, either in equilibrium or in motion; what could be loosely translated as "specialized stretching." This stretching technique was the basis of Greek athletic training.

The term *tension* is also used of the elastic force of gas or vapor. Scientists have discovered that a muscle in action generated a greater elastic force which produces movement. In a steam engine the elastic force of a gas, generated by fuel combustion, is converted to energy or "work"; this is much the same process as that which occurs in our living tissues.

One of the effects of achieving the condition of tension is a feeling of lightness—almost a sensation of having overcome the pull of gravity—which helps to make movement easy and pleasant. This could be because the upward stretch of tension is counteractive to the downward pull of gravity. This downward pull, I believe, affects us more than most of us realize. While we are growing the upward thrust of life, which operates in all forms of growth, is the stronger force. When we are past maturity its strength ebbs—unless we have learned how to conserve it. And then, you might say, the earth begins to reclaim our bodies. We bend, we shrink measurably, we wither; just as a plant withers and returns to the ground when the life force which lifted it and enabled it to withstand the drag of gravity is spent.

When the muscles are in a state of perfect tension or "weight," the weight of the body is dispersed along their constantly moving cords, so that no "dead" weight collects at one point, which means that muscle fatigue is almost entirely cut out.

The control center from which this muscular power is generated is the diaphragm. The strength and development of the muscles of the diaphragm conditions the rest of the muscular system; it is the center of gravity from which movement radiates. Madame Clara Novello Davies, mother of Ivor Novello, called the diaphragm "the success muscle." She said that the ability correctly to use and control the diaphragm gave poise and self-confidence and was essential to achievement of any kind.

The waist, or middle of the body, is the crucial area. Here are some of the body's most powerful muscles; those of the diaphragm itself, of the abdomen, and the *latissima dorsi,* the muscles which spread from the spine around each side, forming a natural elastic belt of muscle. But in all too many waists there is no sign of these muscles. The condition, instead of tension, is one of chronic crumpling.

The slackness of the muscles means that the top half of the body subsides onto the hips, very much like a collapsed concertina. This, more than anything else, produces the "middle-age spread." The pressure of weight of the upper part of the body puts an unnatural strain on the hip muscles. They develop disproportionately and the hips lose all symmetry. Greek men and women, as their statues at this period show, had attractively slim hiplines. You, too, can have a Grecian hipline when your muscles have learned to work the Greek way.

HOW TO DO IT

What we are going to do is to learn how to produce a condition of tension, or "stretch," in every muscle of the body, including, by the way, the face.

1ST STEP

Stand in front of a long mirror, with the feet together touching each other. The weight is thrown forward, onto the balls of the feet. The hands, fingers also touching, are stretched down straight by the sides.   •

Now check on your posture. The old rule of being able to draw an imaginary line from the earlobe through the shoulder, hip-joint, and knee down to the ball of the foot if you are standing correctly still holds good. Make sure that you have got this posture right before going on to the next step. If necessary, practice until it comes naturally. It is a waste of time to attempt the rest of the program until you can manage this; you would be likely to use the wrong muscles. And then you would get a condition of tenseness, not tension.

2ND STEP

Having got your preliminary posture right, draw up from the waist, as if you were trying to pull yourself in two. At the same time, press in the muscles; try to make the front of your waist touch your spine, as it were. This pulling-up action lifts the rib cage, and the shoulders go with it. Be very careful not to raise the shoulders separately, so to speak, and keep them well pressed back. Stretch downward with the thighs and legs, so as to exert as much pull against your upward waist movement as possible. Stretch and counterstretch; that is the principle to keep in mind, and the secret of the success of this method.

3RD STEP

Now straighten the neck, pulling it up from the shoulders—which are pressed back, you will remember. Extend the neck upward as much as you can.

4TH STEP

Stretch the arms downward as much as you can, and push downward with each finger, separately. The arm-stretch exerts a counterstretch against the upward pull of neck and shoulders—but be careful that the shoulders are not dragged downward.

5TH STEP

Against the fulcrum of the stretched and back-pressed neck, push the chin a little forward, and lift it slightly, so that you feel a pull on the muscles under the chin. Now lift the muscles of the face. This is not an easy process to describe, but beginning at the chin, it is possible to raise the muscles of the entire face. If you smile, you will see what I mean. The muscles of the cheeks automatically lift when one smiles. That is the muscle movement that with practice you can achieve without smiling—a smile is not necessary to this particular exercise. In fact, it is essential not to smile, because the muscles of the mouth have to do their work, and if the lips were parted, different muscles would be brought into play.

So you lift the muscles of the face, and the mouth goes with them, held almost in a pout, until the top lip curves up toward the nose. The cheeks lift until the eyes appear almost half-closed. Now open the eyes to their widest extent; raise the eyebrows toward the hairline.

6TH STEP

Lastly, brace the muscles of the kneecap by pushing the kneecap back as far as possible. Then rise up on to the ball of the toes. The entire body, from the crown of the head to the tips of the toes, is now in a state of tension, and it is well worth while practicing until you can achieve that condition. If you find it too difficult to cope with the facial tension as well as that of the body to begin with, you can practice the former while sitting down, until you are proficient enough to add it to the general exercise. Remember, you must begin the facial tension with the upward stretch of the diaphragm muscles, and continue with the shoulder, neck, and chin movement. A sagging chin begins to sag at the waist; it is a culmination of deterioration of posture and slack muscles of the whole torso.

When you are practicing "top half" tension, sit erect in a straight-back chair. Press the end of the spine against the back of the chair, and draw up the spine as much as you can—and really draw it up, with energy in the movement. Try, as in the general exercise, to "pull apart" at the waist, and press in the muscles of the diaphragm and abdomen as hard as you can.

The shoulders, which are lifted by the movement, are pressed well back. Press back the neck, and press the chin a little forward; lift it slightly. Now raise the muscles of face and chin. Squeeze up the muscles of the cheeks toward the eyes; squeeze up the muscles of the eyes until they appear only as slits. Squeeze really hard—without causing strain, of course. Now against this pressure, try to open the eyes very wide indeed. This exercises and strengthens all the muscles of the face, eyes, and neck, as well as those of the waist and diaphragm.

This is a natural method of dealing with double chins and crêpey necks, and of "face-lifting" in general. The action of the muscles firms and smooths the skin and reconditions it. Lines under the eyes gradually disappear; the contours of face and neck become firm and youthful again.

And, by the way, I am not describing a beauty treatment which can be skipped by men. The muscles of the face, neck, and eyes are as important, in their way, as those of the rest of the body; they must be kept in trim by anyone who wants to realize a condition of complete health and fitness.

As the diaphragm is the control center of the operation of tension, and as the strengthening of its muscles is a prerequisite of achieving that condition, it is a good plan to practice as often as possible the "stretching" of the diaphragm, pulling the waist up and pressing it in. Apart from its benefit to health (firm muscles support the vital organs), this movement results in a slim, supple waist and acts as a hip-reducer. This stretching is one of the exercises used by Spanish dancers; you may have noticed their slender waists and hips. Many of them spend regular periods each day with arms lifted high above their heads, trying to reach the ceiling, pulling up the body strongly from the waist. You can do this, too, if you wish. It is a way of speeding up results, and a great aid to figure-beauty.

It was through watching Spanish dancers, Indian women water-carriers, and a Circassian dancer that I realized what the principle of "stretching," correctly applied, can do for the human body in the promotion of health and symmetry. It can produce, as I have just mentioned, lovely lines of waist and hip. It made the necks of the Indian women who carried heavy earthenware *chatthis* (vessels) of water on their heads smooth and firm, even when the women were old. It made the hands and arms of the Circassian woman dancer, who stretched and turned and twisted these parts of her body daily, white and smooth and supple as those of a twenty-year-old although her age was sixty.

The principle of stretching can be used on any part of the body to preserve and restore youth. But to get the best results the condition of complete tension must be achieved. I have described the "sitting stretch," which is one of the ways of getting the muscles into practice for this condition. Another is the arm and leg stretch. The best place to do this is in the bathtub, because then the muscles are relaxed. When in that state they carry out, with less effort, demands made on them.

Sit up straight, with the spine pressed against the back

of the tub, and stretch the spine as much as possible—
gently, of course. Never let an opportunity go by for exercising this all-important part; it is your lifeline. A straight,
supple spine is a strong defense against aging.

Having got your spine into position, with particular care
that the "small" of your back makes contact with the back
of the bath, make sure that the diaphragm is drawn well
up and in. During the whole of the exercise, the diaphragm must be kept in that position; the shoulders must
be pressed well back, and the buttocks pressed against
the bath.

Now lift the left leg at an angle of about 75 degrees to
the body. Stretch it as if you were trying to disengage it
from the hip socket. The stretch must bring the muscles
of the entire leg into play; press back the kneecap, stretch
the calf muscles; stretch the foot and, without moving the
ankle, try to bend the foot downward as far as possible,
from the instep. Do not strain. After a moment drop the
left leg, and repeat with the right leg. Then lift the left
leg at the same angle as before, and again stretch in the
same way, but this time try to bend the foot at the instep
over toward you. After a minute or two, relax and repeat
with the right leg.

Now, still keeping the same position against the back
of the bath, and with the diaphragm well squeezed in,
lift your left arm. The shoulders must be kept firmly
against the bath, acting as a fulcrum to the stretching
process, which is carried out by extending the left arm,
hands, and fingers (which must be kept touching), as fully
as you can, in front of you. The stretch must be felt in
each fingertip. Without moving the shoulder, turn the
arm inside out, so to speak, so that the palm of the hand

and the inside of the elbow are facing you. Keep turning until the movement becomes uncomfortable—but do not strain. Then relax. Repeat with the right arm. Now extend the left arm as before. This time, turn the arm so that the palm of the hand is turned away from you. When you can turn the arm no farther, relax. Repeat with the right arm.

This is what one could call a "muscle reveille." It wakes up lazy muscles, and, incidentally, limbers up the joints. Don't forget full extension and stretching of the fingers. At the end of this exercise, double up the fingers, and press them hard against the palms of the hands, with the thumb folded over the bent fingers. Squeeze fingers and thumbs hard. You can do this finger and hand stretching and clenching whenever you have a spare moment. It is a great help toward keeping the hands supple and healthy —and youthful.

And before we leave the bath, a word about how to leave it. Don't depend on hands and arms to do all the lifting of your body from the water. They will have to do a little of the work, but practice lifting and squeezing the diaphragm muscles, and put them and the abdominal and thigh muscles to work on the lifting job. Do not strain, ever. As the muscles strengthen you will find that you are able to get up more and more easily, until finally a slight push with the hands against the sides of the bath is all that is necessary in the way of assistance.

Do not be discouraged if at first your muscles show no sign of obeying you. Usually, once they have been allowed to get lazy, they are opposed to going back to work. They send messages of despair to the brain; "It's quite impossible. This movement can never be done. We are too

weak and the bones are too stiff." Do not believe them.
If you will keep on practicing, day after day, eventually
the movement that you thought out of the question will
just seem to happen. The body has almost illimitable
powers of response; most of us never tap these powers.
Let me tell you of the case of a woman who did make use
of these possibilities.

She was over sixty; she had had very bad rheumatism
and was using my diet scheme and the "tension" exercise.
Then she told me she had decided to practice the Yoga
"perfect pose" because she thought it would be helpful
in reconditioning her knees and thighs. I warned her that
if she did attempt it, she must be very careful not to
strain muscles or to overdo the practice. No Yoga posture,
or "tension," or any other physical exercise should ever
be carried on a second after it has become painful.

After about three months, she achieved the "perfect
pose"; under the circumstances, a triumph of mind over
matter. It is not an easy pose to master even when the
bones and muscles are supple. But she found the trouble
she had taken well worth while; she said her muscles and
the joints of legs and thighs had become supple again,
and that her general health had improved. In the "perfect
pose" the diaphragm is stretched up, the spine stretched
and straightened, the neck is straight and the shoulders
properly poised; and as these physical positions are vital
to health, they could have had a positive effect on her
condition.

You will find that if you adopt this posture (straight,
stretched-up spine, including the neck; correctly held
shoulders, stretched-up diaphragm), you will be able to
survive without discomfort long hours in a sitting posi-

tion, if a long sitting-session is necessary; for instance, a whole day's motoring.

Very soon, as your muscles begin to strengthen and obey you, you will discover how comfortable this condition of stretch or tension is. Your body, instead of being about as manageable as a sack of potatoes, as are most bodies with untrained muscular systems, is under the control of your will. Movement begins to be a pleasure instead of a wearisome and perhaps painful process. You actually feel you want to move, for the sheer pleasure of it, for the sense of well being it produces. And that feeling is not illusory; it is real. Movement of the right kind stimulates glandular secretions. So you feel better, and you are better, and you want to use the body more and more. The body was made for use, so a circle, not of the vicious but of the constructive type, is formed.

But here and now, I would like to remind you of the basic factor, without which full results are not possible—food. The needs of the muscles—as well as, of course, those of the whole body—must be met if they are to work well for you. They need liberal amounts of riboflavin, pyridoxine, and all the B vitamins. They need calcium, and Vitamin E, and the other minerals and vitamins which combine together in the manufacture of the living flesh.

The foundation of any system of rejuvenation, any method of health improvement, must be food—at any rate at our present stage of development. Highly spiritualized types—adepts or yogis—may be able to get all the nourishment they need from the air (in which, as we know, all the elements are in solution) but our bodies must have more solid fare.

This, then, is the secret of bringing back the muscles

to full life—right food, right use. If you will apply these principles faithfully, you will find almost unbelievable changes taking place in your physical being; as I have already said, a very real resurrection of the body will take place.

SUMMARY

ONE OF THE BASIC ELEMENTS in our longevity program was pointed out in Chapter 3: *movement and the proper use of muscles.* Up to this point in the book we have been dealing with the basic factor, *food,* and we shall return to it in Chapter 13 when we examine the all-important aspect of food for the brain. In the meantime let us explore (as we have begun to do in Chapter 9 and continue in Chapter 10) the recipe for rejuvenation contained in mastering our muscles.

Chapter 9 has covered quite simply a procedure for muscular organization—learning to use specialized stretching (*tension,* not tenseness) for our purposes. In Chapter 10 we shall have more of the same.

In Chapter 11 we shall look at the third of our stated essentials, *breathing,* and then combine what we have learned and relearned in the business of relaxation in Chapter 12.

CHAPTER
10

CONTRIBUTION OF YOGA

THE ancient science of Yoga includes in its teachings a
system of postures, or *asanas*. Physically speaking, the
aim of these asanas is to preserve or restore muscular
tone of a very high order, to recondition the nervous and
glandular systems and the organs, and to promote by this
action long life, long youth, and health.

There are eighty-four asanas; it is said that there are
many thousand variants. Some of these are so complicated
that, to Western eyes, they seem to be meaninglessly elaborate contortions. But every twist or turn of limb or muscle
is made because of a calculated reaction which it produces
in some part of the body. Yoga is an exact science.

The science of Yoga has been in existence for at least
two thousand years as a philosophy and way of life. The
physical-training side of it is looked upon as the kinder-

123

garten, but nonetheless valuable, phase. Concerning it, Gheranda, one of the great *gurus* (Yoga teachers), told a disciple: "As by learning the alphabet one can, through practice, master all the sciences, so by thoroughly practicing the physical training, one acquires the knowledge of the True."

Some of the asanas, although they may be elementary to a Yogi, are so difficult for the average Westerner that their use would not be a practical proposition for most of us. But there are a few asanas which can be learned and used by anyone in average health without too much trouble. Their effects on the health and in reconditioning the body are so far-reaching that they are well worth any effort necessitated in acquiring proficiency in them.

Tension and control of the diaphragm, which I described in the last chapter, will help you in carrying out these asanas, because they are an aid to muscle control. A most important point to remember when practicing Yoga—or any form of exercise—is *never strain*. And never hold a posture once it has begun to cause discomfort, let alone pain. Stop at once and relax. Caution is the keyword in mastering these asanas; however slow the response of the body may be, do not force it. Your muscles may be so obstinate that sometimes you will feel that to go on is a waste of time, that you will never make the grade. But nothing is more sure than that you can achieve your goal if you persevere.

ASANA NO. 1

This asana gives suppleness and muscle tone to thighs, legs, and feet and stimulates nervous energy. First, stretch as described in the preceding chapter, so that the spine is straight and fully extended, back, chin, neck, and shoulders correctly poised, waist and diaphragm well stretched up. Now sit on the floor. Bend the legs backward, keeping them close to each side of the body, so that the left heel touches the left buttock and the right heel is against the right buttock. The arms are fully extended; the palm of the left hand is placed on the left knee, the palm of the right hand on the right knee. The buttocks rest on the floor, between the heels.

At the first, you may find it impossible to get into this position. After a little practice, you will be able to manage that much, but you are not likely to be able to stay in it for more than a second. You should aim at holding this and all asanas described in this chapter for some minutes; five, ten, or even twenty, if you wish. Unlike ordinary physical "jerks," which achieve superficial results by sets of movements, the incomparably great effects of the physical Yoga practices are brought about through maintaining for a set time the limbs and muscles in certain postures.

ASANA NO. 2

Sit on the floor, having first assumed the "tension" position. Stretch out your legs in front of you. Keeping the diaphragm well stretched up and the waist squeezed in— but not so much that your breathing is interfered with— bend the trunk forward from the waist, stretching the spine, until your head rests on your knees. Your hands are grasping your ankles, and your chin, first extended, is then tucked in tightly against your neck, in the so-called chinlock. Keep the cheeks well pressed up; do not let them sag. You will find at first that you cannot keep your legs flat on the ground, and probably to grasp your ankles is too great a strain. Bend your knees up until you can touch them with your forehead without too much effort, and if you cannot reach the ankles, clasp the legs a little higher up. The arms should rest on the floor beside the legs. Do not be satisfied with half-measures, however. Every day, try to bend your knees less and to shift your hands down toward the ankles. This asana stimulates the flow of blood to the lumbar and sacral regions; it is strengthening and invigorating, once you have mastered the position and the "pull" on spine and muscles is operating fully.

Let me warn you again not to hurry or force your body, even though you may despair of ever persuading head and knees to meet. Muscles, like Rome, are not built in a day; reconditioning may be slow, but it is sure. Even before you are able to persuade your body into the position you aim at achieving, with practice results begin to appear. This asana warms up the body; it has an excellent effect upon the circulatory system. Its purpose is also to reduce superfluous flesh, and for this I have found it most effective. It also strengthens the digestive organs. You can vary the position slightly when you are proficient, by grasping the toes instead of the ankles and by resting the forehead on the thighs.

ASANA NO. 3

The shoulder-stand has been called the "king of the asanas." Lie down flat on the floor on a mat or carpet. The

entire length of the spine, from its base to the back of the
neck, should be in contact with the floor; the legs must be
kept stretched out. This is, in itself, a spine-straightening
and stretching exercise, and at first it is unlikely that you
will be able to assume the posture. The area which usually
needs particular attention is the small of the back, where
the spine tends to arch away from the floor. Press it well
down, but take care that the rib cage does not then rise
unnaturally (you can press it down if it does), and that
the shoulders do not lift in sympathy. The shoulders must
be in firm contact with the floor. Hands and arms are
stretched out straight by the sides of the body.

What you are aiming to do in the shoulder-stand is to
raise your body straight up, so that the trunk is at right
angles to your neck and head, which, with the exception
of your arms and shoulders, are the only parts of your
body on the ground. The chin must be firmly tucked into
the neck, and the muscles of the face lifted as described
in the preceding chapter. In this way, muscles of face and
neck are exercised and strengthened. This asana strengthens and reconditions the cervical region of the spine; it
stimulates the flow of blood to this area, and to the brain.
It is valuable to the health generally and a factor in
longevity.

This is not in itself a difficult posture—none is, of those
I have described. The only difficulty is in the weakness of
the muscles and their complete inability, when they are
weak, to do what they are told. As I said at the beginning
of the chapter, one of the objects of the physical practices
of Yoga is to strengthen the muscles. The asanas will do
that, if you are patient and allow the muscles time to re-

condition themselves. You cannot hurry the process; nothing is gained by strain.

If, to begin with, you find you cannot raise the body at all, which is more than likely, you can lever yourself up by means of a chair, a bed, or some other solid article of furniture. Do not stay in the position for a moment longer than is comfortable. Rest for a few moments, then try again. Three such attempts are quite enough for your first few practices of the asana.

ASANA NO. 4

The entire spinal cord is bent and stretched by this asana, which stimulates the flow of blood to the dorsal and lumbar region. It helps to strengthen the digestive system and to promote healthy bowel action. It must be carried out with great care; you must not attempt to do more than you can carry out with comfort. Lie flat on the floor, as for asana No. 3. Raise your legs, but instead of lifting them in a straight line, as in the shoulder-stand, bend them forward over your head until your toes touch the ground behind your head. Hands and arms are stretched out on the floor on either side of the body as for the shoulderstand.

This asana is a superb method of stretching the spine, and spine-stretching is of the greatest importance to health and long youth and long life. Even though to assume the posture may not be possible for some time, each practice is helpful in making the spine more supple. Always stop immediately you feel you have gone far enough in this exercise, and always rest before you repeat it. One or two attempts at a time are enough to begin with.

ASANA NO. 5

The head-stand, the completed inverted posture of the body, is the asana most people associate with the practice of Yoga. It is considered an important item of the physical training of the Yogi; from our point of view, it has great practical value. The reversal of the blood flow in the in-verted position is as good as a holiday for the blood vessels and for the muscles of legs and thighs, which get a chance to relax as probably they never have before. A flow of blood is stimulated to face and neck and head, which means that the important glands in that area are extra-well fed. The hair and the eyes also get their bonus of nourishment. In the Hatha Yoga Pradipika, it is said: "After six months of practicing [the head-stand], wrinkles and gray hairs are not seen."

The inverted position helps to strengthen eyes and eye-sight; the nervous system benefits and the calming effect on the mind is well known. I have been told that eminent statesmen in Pakistan and in India use the head-stand regularly every day, and one, at least, of these men lets nothing interfere with this practice. On one occasion, a very important visitor had to wait because it was the time for Mr. X's *sirsasana* (head-stand), and he could not be disturbed. One of the effects of sirsasana is that it gives a great feeling of wellbeing and vigor—and of being able to cope with any person or situation.

The method of carrying out this asana is to kneel on the floor, bend the head, and place the forehead on a small, flat pad or cushion. Clasp the hands around the head, lac-ing the fingers together to form a support for it. The fore-arms rest firmly on the floor. This is Position 1.

Position 2 is the vertically raised trunk, but with the legs still bent back against the thighs. Position 3 is the fully inverted body. To begin with, weak muscles simply will not do the job of raising the body. In the meantime, in order to practice the exercise and to get the feel of the inverted position, kneel in front of a solid piece of furniture which will support your shoulders and which is close enough to a wall to enable you to climb up that wall with your feet. The result will be a slanting position, in which you can practice taking away first one foot and then the other from the wall. This will enable you to train yourself gradually to do without support.

Now lower yourself gently to the ground. Kneel with your forehead supported on your clenched fists, placed one on top of the other, for a few moments. Never get straight up from the inverted position; you must give your body time to adjust itself. Do not do this exercise more than once at a time until you are completely used to it; even then, twice will be enough until you are really proficient. It is *absolutely necessary* to rest for a short time and to relax between asanas. The best way to do this is to sit in one of the positions of Yoga; the easiest of these is a simple cross-legged position in which one foot is under each thigh. I have come across several variants; one of which is to cross the legs at the ankle with the thighs flat on the floor, forming an angle of approximately 75 degrees with the body. The right foot rests against the body at the crotch, with the toe tucked between the calf and the thigh of the left leg. The left leg is under the right leg, the heel is slightly under the crotch, and the foot against the right thigh. When your muscles are trained and supple, you might prefer to use this position, which is more

restful than the easier one. The most difficult of the three
is the Lotus posture or *Padmasana*. In case you might like
to try it later on, I will describe it. As you can imagine,
these sitting postures make the muscles of the legs, thighs,
and feet supple. They help to slim the ankles and to make
walking easier.

Sit on the floor, as always with the spine straight, the
diaphragm drawn in—and up—and the muscles of the
abdomen drawn in. Chin and shoulders are in the position
described for the other postures. Extend both legs fully;
feel the stretch of the muscles as in your "muscle reveille."
Now place the left foot on the right thigh. You will find
that it is helpful to support the ankle with one hand;
with the other gently press the knee toward the floor. Do
this while you count ten, not with a continuous pressure,
but rhythmically with each count. Stretch the leg out
straight again and relax. Now do the same thing with
the other leg. When you can keep the knee of each leg in
turn on the ground after your foot is in position on the
thigh, raise the knee of the stretched leg, still with the
other foot on the thigh. Do this with each leg several times.
When you find you can keep the thigh of the crossed leg
flat on the ground, you can attempt to cross both legs so
that each foot rests upon the thigh of the other leg.

These exercises firm the thighs and legs and make them
supple. Flabbiness disappears; the skin is reconditioned
and regains its smoothness.

MUDRAS

Mudras are another aspect of Yoga physical training; they
could be described as asanas plus action. I am going to

tell you about one of them, because it does wonderful
things for the muscles of the abdomen and diaphragm—
and, as you know, these are the key centers of physical
fitness. According to Yoga texts: "The practicer of this
[mudra] if old, becomes young again." And: "By practicing this [mudra] for six months, one can undoubtedly
conquer death." I think that to achieve these rather
comprehensive ends through the practice of mudras, one
would have to become a Yogi in earnest, which would
mean altering our way of life more than most of us would
wish to do. For the purposes of this book, I think it is
enough to look upon the practices I have dsecribed as a
series of physical exercises, with much more far-reaching
benefits than the ordinary run of physical "jerks" could
give. And because they do produce these effects, even
when used out of context of the ancient science, they can
make a handsome contribution to our efforts toward longevity.

Here is the mudra. Stand with feet apart, knees bent,
hands on thighs, wrists a little down, elbows pointing out-
ward. Get comfortable, then exhale all air from the lungs.
Now draw up the abdominal muscles and contract them
as much as possible. Now relax. Repeat without taking
another breath, if possible. Do this two or three times
without breathing in. Then relax, and breathe deeply for
a few moments. Before beginning the exercise, the spine
should be straight and the shoulders in their correct position.

The full-dress Yoga practice of this mudra would entail
contracting the abdominal muscles so strongly and raising
the viscera so much that a hollow would be formed under
the diaphragm—a hollow so large that both fists could be

placed in it. I think you will find that a much milder form of this exercise is enough to accomplish what we want, which is the strengthening and toning of the abdominal muscles and those of the diaphragm, and massage of the internal organs.

There are some general points which should be kept in mind concerning the practice of Yoga exercises. They should be done when the stomach is empty and in a warm room. Apart from these provisos, choose the time and place which suits you best, so long as you do not leap out of bed and at once begin exercising.

No asana should be held for more than ten seconds to begin with, and not for so long if pain or discomfort is felt. Each asana can be practiced for about five minutes at a time as a beginning (constantly adopting the position and relaxing during this time), so long as no strain is felt. Later, extend the time as you feel inclined.

Never, never tire yourself or allow any strain or pain. All Yoga practices are designed to strengthen, and to increase vitality; a process which cannot be hurried. You will find you have made progress on most days if you do not overtax your strength—but sometimes you will feel that you are worse than you were the day before. I do not know why there should be this appearance of backstepping; it seems to operate when one is learning any technique, as you no doubt have noticed. It is apparently impossible for most of us to advance in a straight line—so do not lose hope when your muscles seem to be more intractable than they were to begin with. They must—and will—obey you in the end.

CHAPTER

11

BREATH OF LIFE

THE first thing we do when we come into this world is to breathe. It is the last thing we do before we leave it. And, in the meantime, breathing is the most important of all functions of the body. We can live days without water, weeks without food, only seconds without air.

Air is our main source of oxygen. And the body needs more oxygen than any other element. According to Clarke's estimate, the chemical composition of the body is 65 per cent oxygen. It is a kind of maid-of-all-work of the system.

Oxygen enables the body to throw off impurities; it is essential to the functioning of the muscles—and that includes the heart, which is the most important muscle of all. The brain is greedy for oxygen; its cells must have oxygen and then more oxygen, so that they can do their

complicated work. The brain cells deteriorate and die
without oxygen more quickly than those in any other part
of the body. You could say that oxygen is consciousness;
only brain tissue which is oxygenated registers consciousness and is sensitive. The more oxygen we have, the more
lively and aware we feel.

In fact, oxygen is the great source of energy. But you
can have too much of a good thing, and you can get drunk
on oxygen. Which is not to be recommended—any more
than it would be a good idea to have an oxygen inhaler
and keep treating yourself to whiffs from it, as Mr. Yul
Brynner told Mr. Roderick Mann that he did, according
to a report in the London *Sunday Express*.

The best way to get oxygen, unless your doctor pre-
scribes inhalations for some special need, is from the
atmosphere in the usual way: by breathing, of course. But
there are many methods of breathing, some of which enable us to make better use of the air than others.

Yoga rates breathing as a science in its own right. Some
of the Yoga techniques of breathing are so complicated
that few of us would have the time to master them even
if we wanted to. Some of them are easy to learn and to
use, and their results are far-reaching in benefits. They
can be used to improve the circulation, calm the nerves
and the mind, inhibit pain (headaches and even tooth-
ache), or to generate energy. Yoga teaches that correct
breathing can rejuvenate the body and increase the life
span, that it improves the health of mind and body. So
it is a "must" for us.

Here are two basic breathing techniques for inclusion
in the longevity plan. They help to build up vitality and
general wellbeing; they take up very little time. You can

practice them night and morning, before you go to sleep (which, incidentally, correct breathing helps to induce), and when you wake up.

The first is the *complete breath* and is a form of rhythmic breathing. Both points are important—the completeness and the rhythm. We will take the first point, complete breathing, to begin with.

Not many people think about breathing; they just breathe. And the action is shallow; that is to say, the lungs are not expanded, as a rule, to anything like their full capacity. When you have mastered the complete breath, you will be able to get full benefit from the air.

You can breathe completely, sitting or standing or lying, but I think you will find the easiest way to learn how to do it is to practice in a lying position.

Lie down flat on a comfortable bed or sofa. No pillows, no belt, or any form of constrictive clothing around the chest or midriff. To begin with, forget about breathing. Put your hands on your abdomen, and push them out with the abdominal muscles as hard as you can. Now transfer the hands to your ribs. Again, try to push the hands away with the ribs. Do the same thing with your chest. Be careful, while doing this, to keep your shoulders in place; they must not rise toward your ears.

When you have mastered this first step, repeat the process, this time breathing in, imagining that you are pushing your hands away with your breath. Draw the air in deeply, especially as you finish the exercise, so that the tips of the lungs—which quite often get left out—are well filled with air.

Breathe out gently, and as slowly as you can, without straining.

When you can manage this easily, repeat as before, but now put a finger on your pulse, and breathe in to the beat of your heart. Take note of how many counts you make while filling up with breath. Try to hold the breath (when the lungs are full) for half that number, then breathe out for the same number of counts as you breathed in. At first, the number may be ten or even eight counts. Gradually you will be able to increase the total, but never strain the lungs either in overfilling or in holding the breath too long.

When you have completed the exhalation—and in order to get rid of the last trace of air, press in the abdomen as hard as you can—hold the lungs empty for half the number of counts to which you breathed in; then begin breathing in again.

When you can do this exercise easily, you will find that the rhythmic breath charges you up, as it were. If you are nervous or tense, it brings relaxation. The whole body vibrates like a dynamo to the rhythm of the heartbeat, and this gives an indescribable sense of wellbeing and vitality.

At the end of any breathing exercise, always use the cleansing breath, which rests the lungs. This is how it is done. Breathe in, using the complete-breath method; then expel the air from the lungs in a series of short, sharp puffs through pursed lips, as if you were whistling.

The second of the two techniques about which I spoke is the alternate-nostril breathing. You use the complete-breathing method, rhythm and all, but this time you inhale through the right nostril only and exhale through the left nostril. Then inhale again through the right nostril, and so on. The Yogis have a ritual way of closing the nostrils. This is done by bending the first and middle finger, first, against the palm of the hand. The thumb is used to close one nostril, and the third and little fingers to close the other. I am sure that the instructions to use specified fingers have some significance, because, as I have said, Yoga is an exact science, but from our present point of view I do not think it would matter very much if you found it easier to use, say, the thumb and first or second finger for the nostril-closing. Repeat the exercise, inhaling only through the left nostril, exhaling only through the right.

A variant, which you can use as well as the form of breathing just described, is to inhale (according to previous instructions) through the left nostril (while the right is closed), hold the breath, then exhale through the right nostril while the left is closed. Hold the breath and repeat, inhaling through the right nostril and exhaling through the left. Then inhale again through the left nostril, exhaling through the right nostril, and so on.

When doing this exercise, use the chin-lock, which means that during the suspension period between exhaling and inhaling, the chin should be pressed firmly into the neck, the jugular notch. If you press up the muscles of the face at the same time, this is very good exercise for them. And it works wonders with the glands.

Always take great care not to let the breath rush out fast when you are learning these techniques (or at any time) and, I repeat, never, never strain the lungs.

You will find that these exercises help in the control of the nerves and emotions. When we are angry and upset, the breathing quickens; if, at such a time, we consciously begin to breathe deeply and rhythmically, the storm subsides as if by magic. It works in any crisis, any awkward situation in which you feel the need of "plus" to enable you to cope.

These techniques which I have described enable you to make use of the breath of life so that it becomes the breath of long life.

SUMMARY

BREATHING is the most important of all functons of the body. It is also essential number three in our program for long youth and long life.

Here are two basic breathing techniques for inclusion in the longevity plan.

- complete breath—rhythmic breathing: both factors are important, completeness and rhythm
- alternate-nostril breathing

CHAPTER

12

RELAX AND LIVE LONG

To be able to relax is one of the secrets of living—long, successfully, or any other way—and of success in any achievement. Lovelock, the celebrated athlete, once said that this was the secret of his endurance and speed. He was most relaxed, he said, when running his fastest.

"Rest in action" is the power that puts and keeps us on top of our form. Anyone who plays golf knows the havoc that pressing causes. It is the same with tennis or any other game. In every field of endeavor, what we are trying to do or be is likely to elude us if we get keyed up.

When we are tense we cannot see clearly, mentally—or physically. Tenseness disturbs the mental processes. It upsets the functioning of the eye muscles. It exhausts energy, generates poisons in the blood—and so ages us. In fact, tenseness throws a spanner into the whole works.

You know the saying *More haste, less speed?* Trying to rush things make us tense, so it is likely we shall bungle whatever we are hoping to do. There is another tag which shows a better way to handle a situation: *Festina lente* (make haste slowly).

Hospitals, nursing homes, clinics, and psychiatrists' waiting rooms are full of people who cannot do that. And not only in Great Britain. The Royal Bank of Canada not long ago turned over the whole of its monthly letter to what it called "the problem that bedevils every adult person in Canada," the problem of tenseness. The Bank letter described the situation in these terms. "We are victims of a mounting tension; we have difficulty in relaxing. Our high-strung nervous systems are on a perpetual binge. Caught up as we are in the rush all day, every day, and far into the night, we are not living fully. We must remember what Carlyle called 'the calm supremacy of the spirit over its circumstances.' "

A Washington official said that in twelve months there was a total of seven and a half million headaches in the United States. He worked that out on the basis of the number of aspirins sold in a year in America—*over 30 million dollars' worth.* The number of headaches averaged out, he said, at fifty per capita per annum. And twelve million doses of sleeping tablets are used every day. We are living in the "Aspirin Age," as it has been called, the "tension age."

In English hospitals at the end of 1948, there were 200,-000 beds for mental illness, against 315,000 for all other types of illness. What put the patients there? In the majority of cases, the fuss and the fume and the fret of life as most of us live it; continual tension; the inability to relax.

Some burden these 200,000 people were carrying became too heavy for them. Breaking point came, mentally, just as it does physically; tenseness works in the mind as it does in the body, more or less—whether its origin is mental or physical, each form of tension will be affected by the other.

Tenseness is dangerous to health because it is only half a process. And if nature abhors a vacuum, she detests half-measures quite as much and insures that there are unpleasant reactions unless a process is completed, as it was meant to be. Natural laws and all life are made up of pairs of opposites: light and darkness, cold and heat, action and reaction, contraction (or tenseness) and expansion (or relaxation), which must work together for completion.

A muscle is tensed—that's according to plan. But if it does not relax properly, that is not according to plan. So things go wrong, acids form. And if the meticulous routine is interfered with too often, serious trouble results.

It's no good arguing with nature—she always has the last word. If we want to keep healthy and live out our normal span, we have got to relax—and there's no getting away from that.

How many people *do* relax these days? Increasingly few, it seems. Look around you, next time you are in a bus or train or restaurant. You will see your neighbors tapping their feet, fidgeting with ticket, gloves, table silver, according to what is handy; fiddling with tie or collar, hat or handbag, according to sex. They are making all these useless movements because the subconscious is trying to relieve (or externalize) tension. Actually, all that happens is that nervous energy is wasted.

And that—depletion of nervous energy—only increases tension. Fidgeting is a luxury no one can afford.

No one can afford tenseness in any form. Yet, as we know by the astronomic sales of aspirin and sleeping tablets, increasing numbers of people are its victims.

Tranquilizers are a current means of "relieving" tenseness. Tranquilizers are drugs which deaden pain, stupefy the nerves, and give an illusory sense of wellbeing. They are likely to become a very grave threat to human health, mental and physical. There are cases in which their use is justified; they can be valuable in emergencies, but they seem to be rapidly becoming a sort of general panacea. They are taken in cases of rheumatism, arthritis, allergies; in all sorts and kinds of complaints.

Most drugs have injurious effects on the tissues, the glands and their secretions—and, through the glands, affect mental reactions, emotions, and character. The Surgeon General of the United States Public Health Service, Dr. Thomas Parran, particularly condemned barbiturates. They make people sleep, certainly. But if they are taken regularly, bad character traits develop and sometimes criminal tendencies. Some British doctors blame potassium bromide for causing insanity, and even call it a killer.

Neither tranquilizers nor any other drug can do more than give a few hours' respite from whatever your trouble may be, and when the effect has worn off, you are likely to find yourself in a state worse than your previous condition. You can't buy relaxation over a druggist's counter.

Nor can you really buy sleep through drugs. Real sleep,

which builds up the mind and rests the whole body, must come naturally, from complete relaxation.

When you are fully relaxed, you are at rest. And then your sleep is deep and tranquil; it recharges you with energy, so that you can cope with your work and with your play without the aid of tranquilizers or pep pills or any other artificial bolstering up of morale.

The trouble is that so few of us are relaxed, by day or by night. And so tension mounts in mind and body, each acting and reacting on the other.

A vicious circle . . . the stress syndrome.

The way to conquer it is by relaxation. *Relax—let go— take it easy.* But how can it be done?

It's a two-way answer, mental and physical. The needs of both mind and body must be supplied in order to solve the problem. And the best way of tackling it is to begin on the physical level.

Supplement the balanced diet outlined elsewhere in this book with massive doses of all the B vitamins, including, in particular, Vitamin B_1 (thiamine), Vitamin B_6 (pyridoxine), and also Vitamin E. Step up your calcium intake with calcium in biochemic form, and also Vitamin D. At bedtime take a nightcap of black molasses and milk, and calcium.

You are now supplying your nerves with their special diet items, which will help them to regain health and normality. You will find it easier to relax when the nerves are well fed.

Systematic relaxation of the muscles also helps the mind to relax. Take every opportunity you can find of "letting go." There will be many—but never too many. When you are traveling, sit so that your spine is fully supported all along its length by the back of the seat. Get your legs into as comfortable a position as possible, with feet close together and parallel. Now let the ground take the weight of your legs. Rest your hands easily in your lap, loosely clasped if you wish. And let your lap support the weight of your arms. Press your shoulders against the seat-back (if this is possible); let it also support the head. One of the secrets of efficient resting is to find support for your head whenever possible. The head is one-twentieth of the entire body weight—a heavy load for the neck and spine to carry for so many hours out of the twenty-four. Give these parts of your body a holiday whenever you can, and see how much fresher and more rested you feel afterward.

When sitting in a chair (the position should be as described in the last paragraph), slip a small cushion into the hollow between shoulders and head, supporting the neck.

Before you get into bed, at least until you can "untense" easily, it is a good idea to use a muscle-relaxing technique. Stand up straight in the tension—not tense—position. Your arms are hanging straight, but not stiff, at your sides. Flick the fingers with a sharp staccato movement, then let them drop. Do the same with the hands and the wrists. Tense the arms at the shoulders, then let them go limp. Wobble your head on your neck, with the movement you use to ease a cork out of a bottle. Then let the muscles relax. Droop forward from the waist, relaxing abdominal and back muscles. Relax the muscles of the buttocks and thighs. Now droop a little farther till your fingers touch the floor, the head drooping with the arms. If you cannot touch the floor easily, do not attempt it at first—but practice until you can manage to do it. In the meantime, just droop as far as you can in that direction. Let your knees and legs sag; flop to the ground, as if you were a bundle being dropped by someone. If you are really limp you won't feel the bump. In any case it would be slight, and a little practice will enable you to make contact with the floor quite comfortably.

Now pick yourself up and immediately get into bed, which should be firm, not yielding—and, above all, not the modern version of a feather mattress, that abomination from the health point of view. Coverings should be light but warm, and if you want a hot-water bottle, have one. You can't relax when you are cold.

Windows should be open to some extent at top and bottom, because that is the best way of making sure of ventilation. But there is no need to fling them wide in cold weather and let in half a gale. That will not help relaxation, either.

When you are snug in bed—only one pillow, please—first lie easily on your back. The organs then adjust themselves in their correct positions.

Imagine, "feel" your body to be as limp as a dishcloth. Then imagine yourself lifting your left leg until it is at right angles to the body. Picture this very clearly. Then imagine that it drops away. It vanishes; it is gone. Do this with the right leg, then with each part of the body. In imagination, stretch the trunk upward, away from the hips; then it, too, is dropped away. The arms are raised (mentally) above the head, then dropped. Neck and head are treated similarly. In this way, consciousness is withdrawn from the body.

An an alternative, use a suggestion technique. Let the mind travel slowly over each part of the body, beginning with the head. Say to yourself: "My mind is relaxing. My brain relaxing. The muscles of my head, my forehead, face, neck, shoulders, are relaxing." Continue in this way down to the tips of your toes. Then say: "I am completely, completely, completely relaxed. I can think of nothing but deep, refreshing sleep. I am getting sleepier and sleepier. I cannot keep awake."

Now turn over on your right side, with the right knee drawn up slightly. Cross the left leg over the body so that it touches the right side of the bed. This rests the spinal column and relieves it of strain

The Yoga postures and the stretching exercise will help to promote relaxation. But in order to make a complete job of it, we must work directly upon the mind as well as the body.

All you need for the practice of mental relaxation is a place in which you can be alone and undisturbed for ten or fifteen minutes, a comfortable chair or daybed—and yourself.

First of all, get comfortable. Relax your muscles by suggestion, as described above. Instead of telling yourself you are getting sleepier and sleepier—you might suddenly find it was tomorrow if you did—say: "I am resting. My mind is resting, my body is resting. I am completely relaxed." Your body will obey you, and your mind will obey you. The mind can only give attention to one thing at a time; if you concentrate on relaxation and don't let your thoughts wander, your mind must relax.

Now imagine that you are draining your mind, just as you would a sink, of all the hurts and worries, resentments, frustrations, and problems which beset you. They are flowing away like a dingy tide. If you imagine this strongly,

you will soon feel a sense of relief, as if a physical pressure
were lifted. While you imagine the outgoing of your difficulties, suggest to yourself that they are draining away.
Now imagine—and suggest—that strength and optimism,
courage, happiness, any quality you need, is surging into
your mind in place of the stale, destructive thoughts. Picture this happening—most people find that to visualize a
flood of light is the easiest way of doing this—feel the ex-
pansive influence of constructive mental qualities.

You can practice rhythmic breathing while "draining"
your mind. It helps the process along in every way.

Don't pass up this technique as childish and not worth
trying. It is a method of influencing the subconscious; it
can do a great deal toward resting the mind and keeping it
healthy, as people who use it soon discover. A regular
draining off of unhappy thoughts sets the mental powers
free to cope with whatever situations may need attention.
And it is amazing, when our minds are cleared in this
way, how many mountains shrink to molehills.

Drain your mind regularly before you go to bed. Then
say to yourself, several times before you go to sleep, that
you are turning all difficulties and problems over to the
subconscious, and you know it can find the answers. The
subconscious is much better equipped to "put two and
two together," as it were, than is the conscious mind. So
if you think out clearly and objectively all the features of
your problem, as if it were someone else's, and then tell
the subconscious to get to work and solve the problem, it
will. But on no account try to worry out the solution consciously, in bed.

It is essential to leave all difficulties outside the bed-
room door—and on the mat outside the dining room. If

you put worry on the menu it is as bad as eating poison with your food. Worry upsets the machinery of the digestive system; acids form. And then all the signals in the system are set for danger.

If you can manage it, take a few moments off to relax (you know the technique now) before a meal. It will pay dividends in terms of improved digestion and in enabling your system to get the full amount of nourishment from the food you eat.

And whenever you have five or ten minutes to spare, you know what to do with the time . . . relax.

Get the relaxation habit. It will do wonders for you; it smooths the way toward a longer life span. It helps you to do what Alexis Carrel said we all must do before we can live successfully—make peace with ourselves.

SUMMARY

RELAX—and live!

You have now seen that you can relax by giving attention to systematic relaxation and by learning how to go about it. You have also seen that there is interaction among proper use of muscles, correct breathing, and relaxation.

Review the practical hints for relaxing the body—and the mind—given in this chapter and put them to use.

And check your diet! Supplement the balanced diet with massive intake of the complex (particularly B_1, B_6), Vitamin D, Vitamin E, and calcium. Make your nightcap black molasses, milk, and calcium.

CHAPTER

13

FOOD FOR THE BRAIN

IF the brain is to keep in good running order for 180 years, it must be well fed and well looked after. Like other parts of the body—the glands, for instance—it has its own special food requirements. The brain is an unbelievably complex and—to us—very precious machine. To it, to a great extent, we owe our survival and our biological supremacy.

We have always lived by our wits, biologically speaking. And we got to the top of the evolutionary tree because we specialized in brain development and outsmarted our relatives, who hadn't got so much to think with as we had. Look at the dinosaurs, the plesiosauri, the ichthiosauri, and other lines in Life's Outsize Department. They went in for bulk, not brains. So smaller fry, better provided with gray matter, made rings around them in the matter of food supply and living conditions. In the end mastery went to the species which developed the "mostest" in the way of brain and developed it most quickly—man.

Now we are struggling for a different kind of survival; to survive for our full life span, to which we are biologically entitled, free from the infirmities and indignities of senility. And, as in our earlier struggles, we still depend for victory largely upon the cooperation of the brain.

The brain is the director of operations. In a sense, the other organs function to provide the brain with the fuel it needs for its activities. But the brain, the dictator, is just as dependent upon its servants for its wellbeing as they are upon the brain for its directives. If the servants go on strike, the director is immobilized; if the director is incapacitated, the servants suffer.

Just as the human species won leadership through specialization, so the brain won control of the other cells by the same process. Every collection of cells (the organs) specializes in some activity which in our earliest ancestor, protoplasm, was general to the entire organism; sex, movement, breathing, and the other functions. The brain cells have become specialized in the "survival" processes; the ability to adapt to and control (as far as possible) environment. They have done this by developing the faculties of remembering, learning, coordinating ideas, solving problems.

The family tree of our organs goes back to humble beginnings. For instance, the very complex mechanisms which you are at this moment using, your eyes, originated in a sort of specialized skin spot. Modern biological chemistry has discovered parallels between the basic actions of the brain—remembering, learning, coordinating—and the behavior of certain fatty substances such as linseed oil. This oil reacts to ultraviolet light in a way which could be described, chemically, as "learning," "forgetting," and "remembering." Linseed oil is similar to fatty substances of which the brain has the greatest amounts, the phospholipids; it is thought that the chemical reactions of the phospholipids ("remembering," "learning," "coordinating") could be the origin of the human brain, which is the most complicated of nature's productions to date. An "electric-brain" scientist told me that enough complex machinery to fill three large rooms would be necessary in order to reproduce even the simplest human brain activity.

The status of the brain from nature's point of view is shown by the way in which its wellbeing is looked after. The ductless glands act to keep it at more or less an even temperature and fixed blood chemistry; it has three different sets of circulation. Each of these can keep the brain cells in action.

And as for the brain's diet, one of the main points is to make sure that it gets a supply of unsaturated fatty acids, because of their predominance in the phospholipids of the brain, as mentioned a paragraph or two earlier, and the probable connection between these substances and cerebral functioning.

Biologists and endocrinologists believe that research will establish the unsaturated fatty acids as one of the important foods for brain cells. Besides their nourishment value, unsaturated fatty acids are considered to be the first line of defense against thrombosis and arterial complaints generally.

Linseed oil, wheat-germ oil, sunflower seed oil and olive

oil are excellent sources of unsaturated fatty acid. As you would expect, brains contain it, also lard and egg-yolk. Feed your brain every day with eggs; put brains on your brain's menu frequently; have an olive-oil dressing on salad, and take wheat-germ oil or sunflower seed oil after your meals, in any case.

Phosphorus compounds are also found in the cerebral cells. The foods in which phosphorus is chiefly found are glandular organs, wheat (whole), wheat germ, beef, cucumber, soya beans, peas, cod-liver oil, cheese, egg-yolk, mushrooms, fish, oysters, seafoods generally, beans, cauliflower, celery, lettuce. Some items on this list should be eaten daily.

Another great need of the brain is for galactose, which is a compound of milk sugar, lactose. Galactose is important to the nervous system of the brain, and especially important to the growing brain of a baby. Human milk has more galactose in it than cow's milk—nature doing all she can to encourage the human brain's development.

For an adult, or for a child, cow's milks is a good enough source of galactose. Too large a quantity of this sugar might upset our physical chemistry; the quantities of milk we are able to drink would not be likely to provide an excess of galactose.

There is no reserve of sugar in the brain apart from the galactose contained in the fatty compounds; it is dependent for its supply upon the blood circulation.

Sulphur is thought to play a vital part in the functioning of the brain. It is necessary to the oxygen-consuming or "breathing" processes of the cells. Sulphur-containing foods for your menu include egg-yolk, figs, garlic, onions, potatoes, watercress, greens, strawberries, carrots, cauliflower, Brussels sprouts, coconut, cucumber, lettuce, cottage cheese.

Copper and zinc are two more nutrients which the brain needs. Wheat and wheat germ are the best sources of zinc. Copper is found in animal liver and in nuts.

Calcium is another necessity for healthy functioning of the "dictator" organ. Lack of calcium has been found to make children—and grown-ups, too, of course—overimpulsive and hysterically uncontrolled. Calcium is found in milk and cheese, chiefly, in the outer green leaves of vegetables, and in apples, asparagus, apricots, oranges, currants, gooseberries, grapes, cherries, and strawberries.

Add iron and manganese to the list. I have already mentioned the chief iron-containing foods; to save your turning back to look them up, they are white fish, green vegetables, mustard and cress, turnip-tops, liver, kidneys, eggs, watercress, dandelion leaves, shellfish, currants, raspberries, loganberries, yellowstone fruit, all dried fruits, and black molasses.

You can get supplies of manganese from parsley, mint, raw egg-yolk (never eat raw white of egg; it inactivates biotin, one of the B-group vitamins), endives, watercress, olives, pumpkin, nasturtium flowers (very good in salads).

Then there are the "brain vitamins." Vitamin E is considered essential to the cerebellum, the back part of the brain. The experiments which led to this conclusion, made by Pappenheim and Goetsch, were some of the first researches made regarding the necessity of certain types of food for different parts of the brain to enable it to fire on all cylinders, so to speak.

Vitamin E has many important functions to discharge in the system, as we have already seen. Its chief sources are wheat germ and wheat-germ oil, brown rice, eggs, and lettuce. Another reason why it is necessary to the brain is possibly because it is "oxygen-sparing," and the brain uses up a lot of oxygen.

The brain needs a great deal of the Vitamin B complex. Riboflavin (B_2 or G) is named as one of the main vitamin requirements, but thiamine (B_1), Niacin (B_2 or PP), and pyridoxine (B_6) have been found essential to cerebral functioning. These first three vitamins are all thought to be necessary in treatment of pellagra, which is a disease of the brain as well as of the skin. And Dr. Spies believes that pyridoxine must be added, also, for complete recovery from the disease.

Pellagra is regarded as a Vitamin-B deficiency disease. It used to be very prevalent in Lombardy; in its serious form it occurs chiefly in the East—Egypt and India, but in its earliest stages it is probably not so uncommon in the West as used to be thought. Dry, roughened, scaly, and cracking skin are some of the symptoms, with abnormalities of the tongue. In the last stages insanity develops; in Egypt, pellagra is the chief source of mental disorders.

I have given you these details about pellagra because it is an example of the close association between skin and nervous tissue (in this case, in the brain). The nervous tissue is really "specialized" skin; skin which, in the embryo, is turned back to front (or outside in) and then grows certain characteristics of the outer skin of the lowest animals—for instance transmission of impulses.

The fact that brain and skin both need the same elements for their health and normality shows how closely akin they are. And this is also a good illustration of what I said earlier—certain tissues of the body have specialized food needs. They must have liberal supplies of this or that mineral or vitamin in order to work properly; if this substance is lacking in the system, they will register its deficiency more quickly than will any other part of the body.

You can see how essential it is to know what foods the brain needs (and, for that matter, each part of the body), and make sure that it gets a supply so that it can keep working well.

When discussing vitamins in an earlier chapter, I mentioned that, whatever you do, you must not take one of the B complex alone. To do that increases the need of the system for all members of the complex, so in that way a deficiency could be made more acute. The entire group of B vitamins must be used; against that background you can pick out for emphasis the particular member of the group of which you may be short. Yeast is one of the best sources of the complex. To make up the riboflavin quota, eat broccoli, cabbage, kale, fresh peas, apples, almonds, green beans, potatoes, eggs, beef, liver, tomatoes, wheat, turnips, cheese. And drink milk. The trouble about milk is that, as I mentioned earlier, riboflavin is sensitive to light. By the time our milk has stood around for some hours in clear glass bottles—or for days, perhaps—"fresh" milk doesn't exist any more. A good deal of the original riboflavin content is not there. Probably about half has disappeared.

Denmark is a jump ahead of us here. The Danish Dairy Organization has awakened to the daily daylight robbery of riboflavin that goes on from clear glass bottles. All milk is now delivered to Danish doorsteps in brown bottles. This is quite a contribution toward improving the national health standard; we cannot afford to waste any of the riboflavin content of our food. Other countries, too, ought to have made the use of amber milk bottles compulsory long ago. The dairies and national Ministries of Health need prodding into following the Danes' progressive steps.

Thiamine, which is particularly essential to the functioning of riboflavin, is found chiefly in whole-wheat bread and flour, and in wheat germ. Barley, oats, beans, and asparagus are also sources of this vitamin.

The fourth member of the B family of vitamins which the brain needs especially, pyridoxine, is contained in wheat germ, liver, milk, egg-yolk, and brewers' yeast.

Above and beyond its special food requirements is the brain's demand for oxygen. It uses more oxygen per minute than any other part of the body; it withdraws from the air in an hour more than its own weight of oxygen. And that is a record, so far as the other tissues are concerned. The cells of the brain need all this oxygen merely to keep alive.

The brain must have this relatively enormous amount of oxygen because it has a higher rate of metabolism than any other tissue of the body. Its unsaturated fatty acids do not contain much oxygen, so they absorb it with gusto and ask for more. When the brain has all the oxygen it needs, we feel on top of the world; alert and fully alive. That is why reasonable exercise, which causes oxygenation of the blood, gives a sense of wellbeing. The less oxygen there is in the brain, the less alive we feel—and are. If the supply decreases beyond a certain limit, we become unconscious. Six minutes without oxygen damages the cells of the brain irreparably. But then an overdose of oxygen (which we are not likely to get by natural means) is also inadvisable; it produces a state of intoxication. We get optimal amounts of oxygen through deep breathing in fresh air and through exercise. Some foods yield oxygen; among these are potatoes, parsley, mint, horseradish, radishes, onions, tomatoes.

Oxygen is used by the brain to burn the lactic acid which is formed by galactose, or glucose, the sugar in the blood, with the aid of various enzymes, and iron and other metals. More oxygen is burnt when the brain is active than when it is "freewheeling"; the temperature of the active brain is higher than that of a torpid brain. When we are asleep, its temperature is a good deal lower than when we are awake; consciousness generates appreciable heat.

There is no reason why the brain should not continue to "combust" and function perfectly for all our 180 years. But it cannot be expected to go on working efficiently unless it is given enough of the right food, as we have seen. Also it must have rest, and it must be exercised. Like every other part of the body, the brain deteriorates with disuse. Like the muscles, the more it is used, without strain (which is abuse), the better it will respond. There are millions of cells, literally, waiting to be called into action. Very few of us make use fully of our brain resources.

It used to be said that the brain began to lose its power at about the age of forty-five, that creative intelligence was hardly present at seventy-five. There is so much evidence now to the contrary that this theory is generally discounted; it never did hold water. At the age of seventy-one, Galileo discovered the rotation of the earth. Titian was ninety-eight when he painted *The Battle of Lepanto*. Several more of his finest works—*Venus and Adonis, The*

Last Judgment, Christ in the Garden—were created after he was eighty. Benjamin Franklin wrote his famous auto-biography after his eightieth birthday. Darwin was over sixty when he wrote a book which shook the scientific world, *The Descent of Man*. His *Power of Movement in Plants* was written when he was over eighty. Gladstone was eighty-six when he made the speech of his life, on the Armenian persecution. The founder of the American Red Cross, Clara Barton, inaugurated the American National Association for First Aid when she was eighty-four. At eighty-nine, she learned to typewrite.

And these examples don't begin to exhaust the list of cases from which I could quote. But the point, I think, is proved. These people can't be written off as freaks; there are too many of them. And what they have done any one of us can do.

I do not mean that we can write immortal prose or verse, or paint a masterpiece; we may or may not be able to achieve flights of genius. I mean that by paying atten-tion to and supplying the needs of the brain, we can help it to function in later—much later—life as well as it does at what is now thought of as the peak period.

We need not grow gaga or senile if we work *with* natural laws instead of against them. It is not just poetic fantasy to talk about the fire of life burning in the brain; it is actual fact. The brain is an efficient combustion unit, and the form of energy it produces is life. The fire will not die down unless we stoke it with inferior fuel or for-get to refuel it.

But that is not the end or the whole of the story. The brain may be dictator of the physical set-up, but it is under the domination of the mind. Complex and mysterious though some of its activities may be, the brain still is only the organ of the mind, which controls it, and through it the rest of the body. The better the condition of the brain, the better the mind will be able to function.

The physical machinery, not only of the brain but of the whole body, must be kept in good running order so that the mind can work smoothly. You would not expect to get a good picture on your television screen if a tube in the set were broken.

SUMMARY

THE HUMAN BRAIN is an unbelievably complex and very precious machine. It has particular nutritional requirements, among them

- huge quantities of oxygen
- unsaturated fatty acids
- phosphorus
- galactose (available in milk)
- sulphur
- copper and zinc
- calcium
- iron and manganese
- Vitamin E
- Vitamin B complex

Consult the Appendix for listings of food sources for these elements.

CHAPTER

14

DOMINANT FACTOR—
THE MIND

A<small>ND</small> now, it is time mind was brought into the picture.

Mind and body act and react on one another; they form a close partnership. But in that association there is a dominant factor; it is the mind.

Even today, few people realize the power of the mind. Metalnikov called it *pharmacodynamic:* it can help us to live out our full biologic span, or it can hurry us off to the cemetery long before we are due there. The mind, like electricity, destroys or creates according to the manner in which it is used.

The mind is always at work on the body. Everything we think or feel, as well as everything that we do, leaves some sort of trace in the physical being. Emotions cause the blood vessels to expand, or to contract, according to their nature. We flush with joy or happiness, we turn white with fear. Bad news has been known to cause sudden death, by bringing about a spasm of the coronary arteries so that no blood flowed to the heart. The glands are affected by our feelings; their secretions increase or decrease with the tempo of emotion. For instance, when we are afraid the vessels of the suprarenal glands dilate. Adrenalin, the secretion of these glands, pours into the blood stream. The blood pressure and the rapidity of the circulation increase.

An unpleasant emotion, if we feel it only once in a while, will not disturb the functioning of the system to any great extent. But if anger, worry, frustration, or any other "destructive" feeling becomes a habit, it can produce changes in the organs and tissues which result in disease. Many doctors believe that the underlying cause of cancer is in the mind; anxiety, resentment, and so on bring about the formation of poisons in the blood. If they become the prevailing mental attitude, eventually the glands and every part of the body is affected. The old saying "Worry kills" is literally true; worry, constant worry, is a deadly poison. It is as lethal as arsenic or cyanide, though it may not act as quickly as they.

Fear has been known to produce dramatic changes in the body. Fear—or shock—can cause skin eruptions, temporary blindness, temporary dumbness. The hair can turn white, sometimes overnight, through fear, in spite of the fact that it used to be said that such a thing was not possible. But when you think of the changes that shock and fright can cause in the blood—a decrease in the coagulation time of the blood plasma, a drop in arterial pressure, a decrease in the number of white corpuscles, we cannot be surprised that the pigment-forming mechanism of the body is affected too. I have seen examples of the "bleaching" action of strain and shock. One was the case of a man whose hair turned pure white just before an extremely serious operation on his ear, at the age of thirty-two. Another case was that of a man who was trapped for several hours on a narrow ledge above a vat of boiling sugar in a jam factory. His age at the time was twenty-five.

Biologists have translated worry and fear and anxiety into the *stress syndrome*. Under its new name, it is as effective a killer as ever; it is thought that the stress syndrome is the basic cause of most deaths, whatever is written on the certificate. We have seen that negative emotions produce states of mind which bring about organic disorders. Stomach and intestines are affected; ulcerations may follow, or colitis and kidney and bladder disorders. All this could be classed as supportive evidence of this theory.

"We die because we think," according to a great biologist. Perhaps we should say "We die because we think wrongly." Bogomoletz says "Man lives—proportionately—half as long as his lesser brethren because he has received from nature the supreme gift—thought . . . because thought, although it exalts when it knows how to discipline itself, slowly, implacably and secretly wears out the body when it is left to its own devices, or to blows coming from outside, blows from men, or blows from Fate. . . . We die too young because (among other reasons) thought uses up our tissues, exhausts our organs and breaks down our cells."

Remember these words of Bogomoletz; they stress the two-edged quality of thought. *It exalts when it knows how to discipline itself;* thought need not destroy our beings with disease or age. When thought is disciplined or directed, it can be a constructive force of which no one knows the limits. The power to think places at our disposal a force of "atomic plus" quality, for good or ill. Of course, in order to get results we must learn how to use that power. And that is not so simple because so few people even know of its existence.

Until comparatively recently, mind was hardly considered "officially" a causatory factor in the health and general experience of an individual. Limelight was centered on the body; even the mention of extra-physical influences was regarded as cranky or freakish, and people who believed in these possibilities were treated as pariahs.

Gradually this attitude is changing. The word *psychosomatic* crept almost unnoticed into medical vocabularies. Now the term, if not its full implications, is accepted by doctors generally. And at last there are signs that the power of the mind is being recognized and utilized.

Operations have been carried out on patients under hypnotic suggestion without anesthetic. Professor Charcot, experimenting with suggestion techniques, found that edema of the arm could be caused in this way. So did Dr. Soubatov, who induced skin eruptions and circulatory disturbances by the same means. Burns and blisters, "suggested" to hypnotized subjects by Professor Posiopolsky, appeared on the skin without application of heat or any other physical stimulus.

The world-famous Dr. Alexis Carrel witnessed phenomena of faith-healing which, according to physiological laws, cannot happen. Dr. Carrel said that most physicians and physiologists deny these "miracles," but "in view of the facts observed during the last fifty years, this attitude cannot be sustained." He lists diseases which have been cured almost instantaneously by extra-physical means. Among these are peritoneal tuberculosis, cold abscesses, osteitis, suppurating wounds, lupus, and cancer. And he notes that "sometimes functional disorders vanish before anatomical lesions are repaired. The skeletal deformations of Pott's disease, the cancerous glands, may still persist two or three days after the healing of the main lesions. The miracle is chiefly characterized by an acceleration of the processes of organic repair."

The opinion of Dr. Alexis Carrel is the opinion of authority. He was an international figure in science and in medicine. I expect you will have heard of his famous experiment with a chicken embryo, by which he demonstrated that life can be immortal, or practically so, under certain conditions. He kept the chicken embryo alive in a test tube for about thirty years. It could have survived indefinitely, he believed, so long as the right nourishment were given and waste products removed. Dr. Carrel also demonstrated the vital part the biophysico-chemical life of the cells, glands, and secretions play in our body.

Dr. Christopher Woodard, a Harley Street, London, specialist, heals by faith as well as by more usual medical treatments. Mr. G. H. Gedge of Bournemouth, England, a faith-healer, has achieved remarkable cures through prayer. I have myself used this power and seen it working. I know a man who had an inoperable cancer which was cured by faith. That was ten years ago, and there has been no relapse. I have seen the medical reports relating to this case; the evidence of X-ray photographs puts out of court the usual explanation made in such cases—that of course the disease wasn't cancer at all.

I have not space here to list even the names of all the healers I know, or of whom I know, or to record the "miracles" many of them have achieved. The total number of men and women working on these lines in the British Isles alone would probably fill a book. The fact that these healers exist and are able to produce positive results in so many cases is described by Dr. Alexis Carrel as "of profound significance." He goes on to say: "Such facts . . . show the reality of certain relations, of still unknown nature, between psychological and organic processes. They prove the unique importance of the spiritual activities, which hygienists, physicians, educators and sociologists have almost always neglected to study. They open to man a new world."

They open to man a new world. . . . This world is the world of the mind; a mysterious, almost unexplored territory, in which scientists now say anything is possible. We have taken a brief glance at some of the results of the powers found in that world. Let us see what has been discovered about its nature.

Einstein, Jeans, Max Planck, de Broglie, and Schrodinger are among the scientists who say that consciousness is the matrix of matter, not matter of consciousness. Mind is regarded by these men as the supreme controlling power of the universe.

"I regard matter as derivative from consciousness," says Professor Planck; "We cannot get behind consciousness." Prince de Broglie's version is: "I do not see how consciousness can be derived from material things. I regard consciousness and matter as different aspects of the same thing." "Thirty years ago," wrote Sir James Jeans in *The Mysterious Universe,* "we thought or assumed that we were heading towards an ultimate reality of a mechanical kind. Today there is a wide measure of agreement that the stream of knowledge is heading towards a non-mechanical reality. The universe begins to look more like a great thought than a great machine. Mind no longer appears as an accidental intruder into the realms of matter. We are beginning to suspect that we ought rather to hail it as the creator and governor of the realms of matter." And: "It may well be that each individual consciousness ought to be compared to the brain cell of a universal mind. I incline to the idealistic theory that consciousness is fundamental. The material universe is derived from consciousness, not consciousness from the material universe." In a later book, Sir James says: ". . . Many of our former conclusions of nineteenth-century science on philosophical questions are again in the melting-pot. There appears to be a case for reopening the whole question as soon as someone can discover how to do it."

Even in the "materialistic" nineteenth century—voices were raised against the limitations of scientific dogma. Professor Poynting said at a meeting of the British Association in 1889: "We must confess that physical laws have fallen off in dignity. No long time ago, they were quite commonly described as the fixed laws of nature, and were supposed sufficient in themselves to govern the universe. Now we can only assign to them the humble rank of mere description, often erroneous, of similarities we believe we have observed."

The only thing we can be sure of nowadays is that—so

far as the conditions under which we live are concerned—
we can be sure of nothing. The general assumption, as
Professor Poynting said, "no long time ago," was that we
had the universe taped, and the cosmos also, at any rate so
far as the broad outlines of knowledge were concerned.
Matter, for instance, was known to be a solid abiding-
place, physically and theoretically.

Now, in the old sense, matter has no reality. Science has
reduced it to indefinable relations between indefinable
parts. As to what matter is, in Einstein's relativity it is
defined as being a form of energy. "Matter is nothing
but motion." Instead of saying "matter has energy," relativity pronounced "matter is energy." And again, "Matter
is the highly concentrated form of the inmost bodily
energy; the energy is hidden so deeply that it seems hopeless ever to release it."

But then, if matter is energy, where does that take us?
Not very far, because no one knows what energy really is.

No one knows what electricity is. No one knows what
radiation is. And no one knows what mind is.

But since matter is thought to be a form of energy, and
since it can be shown that mind acts upon it, it seems probable that mind, too, is a form of energy. Such scientists as
Descartes and Berkeley are agreed that "If mind and matter are fundamentally of different natures, they cannot
interact."

We do not know what energy really is, as I said. So that
to say mind is a form of energy does not explain its true
nature. Professor Joad said that "scientific knowledge is
not knowledge of reality, but only of appearances," and
"At no point have we come within sight of a true explanation, that is, of an explanation which really does ex-

plain. We have only been pushed back to an earlier point in time, the phenomenon which is to be explained. All scientific so-called explanations are of this type. We are only given a slightly more complex and technical account of the fact to be explained."

We may not know what energy in any of its forms actually is, but we know at least something of what it can do and how to make use of it, for instance, in its manifestations as electricity.

And we also can make use of that form of energy which we call mind, scientific consideration of which is so relatively recent.

Physicists who have studied the mind and its activities place no limit upon its powers, and therefore potentially on the use we can make of them. Some scientists not only accept the reality of mind, but rate it as the only reality. Sir Cyril Burt tells us in his *Study of the Mind:* "While the physicist has arrived at the stage when he is ready to assure us that he has a conscious mind, he doubts whether he really possesses a material brain." In other words, he doubts the reality of matter.

Such a statement shows clearly the changing attitude of science toward the mind and its works. Emphasis is beginning to shift from matter to the importance and the potentialities of mind.

The new science of extrasensory perception or parapsychology has helped to establish the empire of the mind. Professor J. B. Rhine, who holds a Chair in Parapsychology at Duke University, North Carolina, is one of the pioneers in this field. He has probably done more than any other single scientist to establish the "reality" of extrasensory powers in general and of telepathy in particular.

Before science began to investigate telepathy, messages of any sort received by one mind from another without physical agency were believed to operate by some sort of "spiritual" transmission service, either from the lower or the upper regions, according to their nature . . . which may indeed be the explanation in some cases, if not in the general run.

Until organized research began, science did not concern itself with an explanation of telepathy. It was considered pure superstition and as such did not rate attention. Many, many years of experiment and a vast weight of accumulated evidence has been necessary in order to make a dent in this attitude, but at last this has happened. In 1949, Professor A. C. Hardy told a meeting of the British Association at Newcastle-on-Tyne that in his belief, "the communication of one mind with another, other than through the ordinary sense, has been established, and that it has passed scientific tests."

Today, telepathy is accepted fairly generally as a scientific fact. And the heat of the argument is turned not on whether telepathy exists but on how it works. The earlier theory of its supernatural nature (at any rate, in most cases), has been discarded. The usually accepted explanation is that telepathy works by some "form of electricity," which is merely a push-back, as Joad said, "to an earlier point in time, the phenomenon which is to be explained."

Professor Rhine thinks that the most plausible hypothesis "would be that the receiver mentally interacts in some way with the sender's nervous system, much as the latter himself does when he remembers something. This would be some kind of clairvoyance, though it might be of a special kind. Or the sender could be operating in some way directly on the nervous system of the receiver, something like the way he operates on his own in bringing about motor responses."

So here we are again: no one really knows what telepathy is. But we do know that it works, which is why I mentioned it. It is another example of the powers of the mind; the powers which act upon and use physical tissue —or matter—for its purposes.

What we are particularly interested in at this moment is the applications of those powers for our purpose; the reconditioning of the body; the prolonging of youth and health and life. We have seen the way in which mind can act upon matter, constructively and destructively. How can we put it to work?

Whatever means we use, the answer is by impressing the subconscious with our desire. There is nothing new about this principle; it has been known for centuries, probably since the beginning of time. Modern science has rediscovered it, and discovered that it works. Its chief techniques—autosuggestion, heterosuggestion, and the controlled use of the imagination—are "rediscoveries" also. They were the basis of magic and witchcraft, probably. The rituals and procedures of voodoo priests, African witch doctors, and Hawaiian kahunas suggest that they made full use of these techniques.

Let us take the method of autosuggestion first. Most of us have heard of Dr. Coué and his formula: "Every day and in every way I get better and better." The phrase had to be repeated over and over again when one was in a drowsy condition, preferably just before going to sleep at night. This is the time when the subconscious is in its most receptive condition, because the conscious mind is at its least active, and therefore least able to repel a suggestion or to argue about its validity.

This Coué formula is an example of autosuggestion; the principle underlying any form of suggestion is the same—that the subconscious accepts as true anything repeated often enough and with enough conviction, if complete attention is given to the suggestion. Suggestion (auto or any other kind) will not produce maximum results— or perhaps any at all—if you are thinking of something else when the suggestion is being made. Suggestion is the "punch" behind advertising and any other form of propaganda. It is one of the strongest weapons of the dictator. Hitler made full use of it.

An accepted suggestion sinks deep into the mind, below the levels of consciousness. You may forget it, so far as you know, but sooner or later it will reappear in the form of an effect, physical or mental.

So what you have to do now is to "sell" to yourself the idea that long youth, long health, and life are possible and possible for you. The way to do this is to make a habit of saying to yourself that every cell of your body is renewing itself, your blood stream is becoming clean and fresh, your muscles strong and supple; that your glands and every organ, every process and function of your body is working perfectly. Construct a short phrase bringing in all these points, and repeat it constantly whenever you have time during the day—when traveling by bus or train, for instance—and always before you go to sleep at night. Fall asleep repeating it; that is the way to get results.

The other technique mentioned, controlled imagination, is the consciously cultivated faculty of image-mak-

ing. It can function apart from, or can be used to rein-
force, the powers of suggestion.

The image- or picture-making ability of our minds is an
important part of our equipment for the success of the
long health and youth and life program. It means the con-
struction in imagination of conditions which we wish to
realize objectively. Constantly repeated exact and vivid
visualization affects the subconscious, and the subconscious affects every cell of the body, so that thought "is
made flesh." The picture which is given to the subconscious to work on must be as clear-cut as possible, and
here again the law of repetition helps. The oftener you
visualize your picture, the easier the process becomes,
and the clearer its details grow. As with suggestion, it is
regular repetition which brings results—and the results
can be amazing.

Let me stress that the pictures constructed in this way
by controlled use of the imagination are not daydreams.
They are the products of a defined technique of creation;
they are "real." They can be photographed. In Paris, Dr.
Baraduct, in a well-known experiment, obtained clear
photographs of images held in the minds of a number of
subjects. The best result was the reproduction of a golden
eagle upon the image of which an ornithologist was con-
centrating. It was found to be exact as a photograph taken
from life. Next best results were pictures obtained from
women in love who were visualizing the men in their
lives. A series of equally successful experiments of the
same type were made in England not long ago.

A point worth remembering before you begin to build
up your *schema* or plan of the physical condition to be
realized is that it is useless to visualize any change in which

you cannot completely believe. For instance, if you are five feet tall and would like to be a six-footer, probably you could not believe that you could grow to such a height.

It is comparatively easy to believe—because it has been proved to be so—that the body is capable of renewing itself and building new health and youth and strength, if it is given the right food and care. The mind's part is to accelerate and increase the scope of this process.

This it can do in many ways. For instance, while you are eating, think of the rejuvenating power which the minerals and vitamins will release in your glands and organs, and imagine this power at work. When you practice breathing according to the methods described, "feel" the life-giving qualities of the air (which, as you know, contain all the elements in vapor form) flooding every cell and tissue; "see" this life filling your whole body as a glowing light. Tell yourself that these things are happening in your body.

Tell yourself you are growing younger and more healthy as often as you can during the day and at sleeptime. "See" yourself constantly as you want to be; believe that every day you are growing more like the picture you have made of yourself. Feel young; tell yourself that every muscle is becoming strong and vigorous, and that to move—to be alive—is a joy. Keep this up day after day.

Perseverance and repetition are two of the chief methods of getting your mind to work for you. And it is worth while making the effort to coopt the powers of the subconscious; they are practically limitless and available to all of us. They can be made use of in many ways—including assistance in managing the Yoga postures.

The method of doing this is to go through the whole exercise in your mind. See yourself doing the movements; feel your muscles carrying them out. You can do this so intensely that the muscles react almost as if they had actually performed the physical movements. This technique has been used by many people, including a famous broad-jump champion. This athlete used to get his trainer to mark out on the ground the distance to be jumped. Then he would lie in a hammock near by, "practicing" his jump mentally. A Hungarian prima donna whom I knew sang at the great opera houses of the world without practicing a note—aloud. She told me that she used to sing her arias over and over again in her mind, "imagining" every note and variation, "hearing" herself singing them. One of the advantages of this method, she said, was that it prevented her voice becoming fatigued. Her husband thought it was a good idea, too.

These are a few examples of what the power of the mind can do for us. But we must not forget that if the mind is to do its best work, it must be properly nourished; just as the body and its organs, including the organ of the mind, the brain, must be given the right food in order to function efficiently. We have discussed the food elements necessary to our physical being; the vitamins and minerals which the mind needs so that it can keep youthful and active, are constructive, positive ideas, "I can" thoughts; plenty of exercise in the way of new concepts and new goals. "The aging of the mind," says Dr. Victor Bogomoletz, "is not the consequence, but one of the causes of the aging of the body. . . . Prolonged youth and long life of the body depend chiefly on the condition of the mind or psyche."

Emerson said: "A man is what he thinks all day long." This is literally true because to think the same type of thought consistently creates an attitude of mind. Eventually this mental attitude affects every cell of the body; it affects the way we move and carry ourselves. So we become what we think; in that sense, we are self-made.

We possess the "supreme gift—thought." And depending upon whether we recognize its power and learn to apply it or neglect it, thought will remake us—or unmake us.

So to learn to control and to use the mind and its powers is a prerequisite of longevity. With the aid of the mind, as science tells us, we can achieve our goal; anything, in fact, upon which we set our hearts—and our minds.

Begin now to make use of this tremendous, immediately and ever-available force. In the words of Metalnikov: "There are no limits to creative power, and the will of man."

CHAPTER

15

SECOND SPRING

THIS can be a wonderful day for you . . . the first day of a second springtime. If you are what is now considered to be elderly or middle-aged, it can be the day you begin to grow young again. If you haven't reached what according to present reckoning is the halfway stage of life (although really it is nothing of the sort) you can begin today to tell old age to wait—indefinitely.

And that is a reprieve, for most of us, from something which, even if we do not dread, we do not look forward to —old age and all that it means: loss of vigor, loss of all the qualities which make life worth living.

No wonder many people say: "I'd hate to live to be 180." They think that an extension of the life span means an extension of the old-age period and its miseries. But the whole point of learning to live to be 180, as you will have gathered from this book, is to learn to prolong not old age but youth and health. To learn to recapture and to keep the energy and eagerness of early years, to discover that these belong to us at any (chronological) age.

In this book, I have tried to bring to your notice the ways, sanctioned by science, past and present, of accomplishing these ends. And to show you that, scientifically speaking, the goal is within the reach of all. I cannot make you young—or happy—or vital. No human being can do that, except yourself. All anyone else can do is to point the way. There is no limit to living, according to science. There is a limit only to the will to live—the limit you set yourself.

The potentialities of living matter are endless. Protoplasm has been proved potentially immortal. We have seen that the life span of animals can be increased by additions and shortened by subtractions of key elements in their diet. And that finally disposes of the previously unquestioned belief that a life span was fixed immutably by natural laws—could be lengthened only by fluke, shortened only by disease or accident.

And as for our own life span, it certainly is not fixed at three score and ten years, perhaps not even at thirty-three score. But at the moment, we need not look so far ahead. It is enough, I think, that we can "tell old age to wait." That is the challenge—and the victory.

The premature aging which we now accept as natural has no part in a reconditioned body—or mind. The body which is given the right working materials will get on with the job of living—almost indefinitely. The mind which is well fed, will continue to function youthfully—almost indefinitely. Let me repeat once more that feeding the mind means feeding the brain (its physical organ) with the right vitamins, minerals, and other nutrients, and also feeding the mind itself with a diet of constructive, positive thoughts which renew and invigorate it. It is just as necessary to sustain the mind in this way as it is to fuel the body with regular meals.

We have to remember also that exercise for the mind is just as important as it is for the body. Planned cultivation of the imagination as described earlier is one way of exercising the mind; the practice of concentration, which is necessary to the success of any organized mental process, is another. And, above all, the best method of keeping the mind healthy and youthful is to have a purpose of some kind.

To work for a constructive purpose is itself one of the greatest aids to longevity. We all know or know of men or women who keep going because they are determined to complete some aim or work. Conversely, there are the people who retire to "enjoy life"—and die within a very short time after retirement because the interest which was the mainspring of their existence is no longer there.

The happiest people are those whose minds and bodies are occupied in reaching some worthwhile goal. So here, as well as the other things we have listed, is an additional "must." Get interested in something if you want to stay alive. Wrap yourself around it; determine to realize your ambition, whatever it is. You can do it, if you make up your mind that you will do it and believe that you can. William James, the great American psychologist, said:

"Our belief at the beginning of some doubtful undertaking is the *one thing that ensures the successful outcome of the venture.*" (Italics mine.)

Perhaps, at this moment, you are saying to yourself that you cannot think of a purpose sufficiently satisfying to be worth the effort of living to be 180. Do not listen to yourself. If you want to live fully and determine to do that, you will find that ideas and opportunities develop in a natural way. They always do, unless we close the doors by saying "There is nothing I can do"; "I can't do this—or that—at my age; I could do it if I were younger." These thoughts are dangerous. They hamstring us; they drain us of energy and the power to do what we would like to do. And they are not true.

In fact there is very little indeed that we cannot do, if we make every possible effort toward achievement and believe in our ability to achieve. Whatever the seeming obstacle may be, "throw your heart over," as athletes training for the high jump are told. You go where your heart goes.

The only reason which could prevent your finding some really satisfying aim for which to work in the next century or so would be to think you can't. That is the same sort of attitude as that which made the children of Israel afraid to advance. "We are as grasshoppers in our own sight," they said. We can never reach any goal, let alone the age of 180, if we see ourselves as "grasshoppers" not able to do what we aim to do.

First cousins to the "grasshoppers" in their mental attitude are the obstacle-hunters. These are the people who, although they would like to live out their full span, and believe that they could do it, worry about what will hap-

pen when. . . . They visualize that world economics and
the whole social fabric might turn topsy-turvy when
enough of us reach the 180 mark.

Our ancestors might just as well have worried—and they
probably did—as to what would happen when the nomad
phase passed into the agrarian or, later, when the feudal
system crumbled. The framework of society has always
adapted itself to the changing pattern of evolution from
which it grows, and it always must, in ways which we may
not always be able to forecast. The social order must
change to conform to our needs, not our needs to conform
to an existing order.

And, touching the economic side of the increased span
of life, we have to remember that as what we now call
"old" people are more and more able to take an active
part in active life, their contributions will mean increased
manpower and increased prosperity.

Nor are we likely to have less in the larder, as some
schools of thought forecast, even if there were a greater
demand on the food supply. It has been established that
the world today could support at least three times its present population.

But the probability is that this question of population
enlarged by the addition of the "100 plus" group will not
arise. It is more likely that nature will adjust these things,
as she generally does, and that as people live longer the
birth rate will decrease. The birth rate goes up and down;
it is a barometer, to some extent registering national needs.
After a war, as we know, it rises, although people in general do not go around saying: "We must have more children." In times of industrial expansion, when manpower

was at a premium, families of sixteen and seventeen were normal. And so history has gone.

And do not let anyone tell you that a rising population is necessarily indicative of racial virility. Much more likely, as we have just seen, it is a matter of expediency or of race-hypnotism, as when Hitler talked the Germans into breeding like codfish.

Nor does a decreasing population inevitably indicate decay. The Greek ideal at the peak of racial perfection was "fit and few," an ideal which we may see realized again in our long lifetime.

Throughout nature, the birth rate is geared to replacement demands of the species. Fish spawn in the hundreds because relatively few of the potential new generation survive the hazards of other fishes' menus and assorted other dangers. Elephants, better able to protect their young, produce only one or two infants at well-spaced intervals.

And, finally, whether we (or anyone else) like it or not, the trend is set for "old" populations. The world of the very near future will be a world with more old people in it than ever before in recorded history. This will mean that we shall be living in a mature society, something that has not existed for many and many a century. Think for a moment of its implications; it has great possibilities.

Most men and women, as they grow older, grow more tolerant and understanding of human problems. And there will come plenty of time in which to study them. Perhaps better solutions of these problems may be found through the wisdom of experience, of which biologists say only a mature brain is capable.

The brain need not decay with age, as we have seen. At

about sixty, which is generally taken as the age of mental maturity, pigment is deposited in certain cells of the brain. This pigmentary deposit is thought of as a symptom of aging but it does not affect the brain's functioning. It seems rather to be an indication of a ripening process comparable to the reddening of the skin of an apple.

Experience teaches. The older age-groups coming into being, who have learned their lessons, will have time to apply them for their own and other people's benefit.

A longer life span will mean, too, a longer span in which the genius of men who have a vital contribution to make to human progress—the Einsteins, Jungs, Darwins, Marconis, and Emersons—can flower fully instead of withering, as now, so much too soon.

I have said that science tells us that there is no reason why we cannot "make old age wait"; I have just mentioned the ability of the brain, the physical organ of the mind, to function almost indefinitely, unimpaired by age. But what about the nervous system, another essential piece of physical mechanism? According to some pundits, that will let us down. Nerve cells as they wear out are not renewed, and there is no known method of resuscitating them. In the face of that fact, how can we refuse to grow old?

It is perfectly true that nerve cells do not multiply, although during their lifetime, as Dr. Bogomoletz tells us, they "undergo a continual process of partial autoregeneration and biochemical adaptation of their protoplasm." Nerve cells die one after the other. But most mysteriously, just as the pigmentation of brain cells does not impair the functioning of the brain, this dying-off does not seem to interfere at all with the mechanism of the nervous system.

It can even work more efficiently in what we now call "old age."

It's just another of nature's paradoxes.

So there is no obstacle, after all, to claiming the 180 years of our birthright, not even the gradual death of the nerve cells. We have the sanction of medical and scientific opinion for relearning to conjugate the verb *to live*, for looking forward to the fresh opportunities and attainments which are open to us by an increased span of health and youth—and life. And of happiness—because there is no point in living to be 180 unless we like it.

But I think that it would be impossible to learn to live long without growing old and not to learn also a technique for full living, which spells happiness. The second spring is the time to fall in love with life all over again, with the interests, experiences, and enjoyments which will come to us unless we shut the doors of the mind and refuse to let them in. It is negative thoughts which we must make it our business to shut out—doubt, fear, apathy, and their fellows. These are among the chief obstacles to reaching the goal of our 180th birthdays—or anything else.

The principles about which I have written in this book work; they can be used by anyone. I firmly and fully believe that you and I have within us everything which it takes to enter into the wonderful experience of a fuller, healthier, happier life, that we can begin to do this now, *at once*, and that we can go on living—and enjoying it—well toward our second century. Always provided we don't walk under a bus, of course. And even that sort of accident is less likely, for many reasons, to happen to a healthy, fully integrated person. But we haven't time to go into that question now.

A second spring-time . . . and it can begin now. Let me wish you many happy returns of the day, in the assurance that they can be most happy. And before I leave you, I want to ask you to a party. It is the celebration of a wedding anniversary of a 24-year-old student of mine. She and her husband are traveling to it by tandem bicycle, she tells me. The date is July 14. The year, 2081. She and her husband will be 150 years old, then. Don't forget, will you? I shall expect you.

APPENDICES
A to H

APPENDIX A

MAJOR FOOD SOURCES OF VITAMINS

VITAMIN A

Butter
Cream
Cream cheese
Kidneys
Lettuce
Liver
Milk

Sources of carotene (precursor of Vitamin A)

Apricots
Broccoli
Carrots
Fish-liver oil
Green vegetables
Kale
Lettuce
Potatoes
Prunes
Tomatoes
Turnip greens
Yellow fruits

VITAMIN B

Black molasses
Brewers' yeast
Milk (dried skimmed)
Wheat germ

Whole-grain cereals
Yoghurt

Sources of B_1 (thiamine, aneurin)

Asparagus
Barley
Beans (dried)
Brewers' yeast
Milk (dried skimmed)
Oats
Whole-meal bread and flour
Whole wheat

Sources of riboflavin

Almonds
Apples
Beans (dried)
Beans (green)
Beef
Brewers' yeast
Broccoli
Cabbage
Cheese
Eggs
Kale
Leeks
Liver
Milk

Peas (fresh)
Potatoes
Tomatoes
Turnips
Whole wheat

Sources of B_6 (pyridoxine)

Brewers' yeast
Egg-yolk
Liver
Milk
Whole-grain bread, cereals, and flour

Sources of nicotinamide (niacin, nicotinic acid)

Black molasses
Brewers' yeast
Milk (dried skimmed)
Soya flour
Wheat germ
Whole-grain cereals
Whole-wheat bread and flour

Sources of pantothenic acid

Black-molasses
Brewers' yeast
Egg-yolk
Kidneys
Liver
Milk (dried)
Peanuts
Whole-wheat cereal

Sources of folic acid

Brewers' yeast
Liver

Source of B_{12} (erithrotin)

Liver

Sources of inositol, choline, beatine

Black molasses
Milk (dried skimmed)
Wheat germ
Whole-wheat cereals
Yeast
Yoghurt

VITAMIN C

Black currants
Broccoli
Cabbage
Cantaloup
Citrus fruits (especially lemons, oranges)
Fruit (almost all fresh fruit)
Kale
Mustard and cress
Peppers (green)
Rose-hips
Tomatoes
Turnip-tops
Vegetables (almost all fresh vegetables)
Watercress

VITAMIN D

Butter
Egg-yolk
Fish (fatty)
Fish-liver oils
Herring
Liver
Mackerel
Milk
Salmon
Tuna

VITAMIN E

Avocado
Egg-yolk
Lettuce
Rice (brown)
Salads (especially lettuce)
Sunflower-seed oil
Wheat germ
Wheat-germ oil
Whole-grain cereals

APPENDIX B

MAJOR FOOD SOURCES OF IMPORTANT MINERALS

ALUMINUM

Widely distributed in foods

ARSENIC

Widely distributed in vegetables and meat

BORON

Most vegetables and meat

CALCIUM

Apples
Apricots
Asparagus
Beetroot
Blackberries
Cabbage
Carrots
Cheese
Cherries
Cucumber
Currants
Eggs
Figs
Gooseberries
Grapes
Green vegetables (especially dark outer leaves)
Honey
Lettuce
Milk
Milk products (except butter)
Olives
Onions
Oranges
Pears
Pineapple
Radishes
Strawberries
Watercress
Whole wheat

COBALT

Eggs
Kidneys
Liver
Muscle meat

COPPER

Asparagus
Barley
Black molasses
Kidney beans
Lentils
Liver
Mushrooms
Nuts

Parsley
Wheat germ

FLUORINE

Drinking water
Meat
Vegetables

IODINE

Artichokes
Asparagus
Beetroot
Berries (dark)
Cod-liver oil
Fish (ocean)
Leeks
Lettuce
Melon
Mushrooms
Onions
Peas (green)
Radishes
Sea-greens (agar-agar, car-
    rageen, Irish Moss)
Strawberries
Tomatoes
Turnips
Watercress

IRON

Beans (lima)
Black molasses
Cabbage
Cabbage (red)
Carrot-tops
Cherries
Coconuts
Currants
Dandelion leaves
Dark green vegetables

Dried fruit
Egg-yolk
Figs
Fish (white)
Gooseberries
Kidneys
Liver
Loganberries
Mushrooms
Mustard and cress
Nettles
Oatmeal
Oranges
Peas
Pineapple
Radishes
Raisins
Raspberries
Shellfish
Strawberries
Tomatoes
Turnip-tops
Watercress
Whole wheat
Yellow-stone fruit

MANGANESE

Agar-agar
Almonds
Egg-yolk (raw)
Endives
Lettuce
Liver
Mint
Nasturtium flowers (in
    salads)
Olives
Parsley
Peanuts
Potatoes

Pumpkin
Walnuts
Watercress
Wheat germ

NICKEL

Most vegetable and animal tissues

PHOSPHORUS

Beans
Beef
Cauliflower
Celery
Cheese
Cod-liver oil
Cucumber
Egg-yolk
Fish
Glandular organ meat
Lettuce
Meat
Mushrooms
Oysters
Peanut Butter
Peanuts
Peas
Radishes
Rice (brown)
Salmon
Sardines
Seafood (generally)
Shrimps
Soya beans
Walnuts
Wheat germ
Whole wheat

SILICA

Artichokes
Asparagus

Celery
Cucumber
Dandelion
Leeks
Milk
Oats
Potatoes (outer skin)
Radishes
Strawberries
Sunflower seed
Tomatoes
Turnips
Whole Wheat

SODIUM AND POTASSIUM
(Biochemic salts)

Potassium found in

Asparagus
Brussels sprouts
Cabbage
Carrots
Cauliflower
Cucumber
Dandelion
Grapefruit
Parsley
Radishes
Tomatoes

SULPHUR

Almonds
Brussels sprouts
Cabbage
Carrots
Cauliflower
Coconut
Cottage cheese
Cucumber
Egg-yolk
Figs

Garlic
Gooseberries
Greens
Kale
Lettuce
Onions
Potatoes
Radishes

Strawberries
Turnips
Watercress

ZINC

Wheat-bran
Wheat germ

APPENDIX C

FOOD SOURCES OF MISCELLANEOUS IMPORTANT ELEMENTS

AMINO-ACIDS:

ARGININE (needed by the gonads)

Eggs	Peanut flour
Milk	Whole wheat
Oatmeal	Yeast

CYSTINE AND GLUTAMIC ACID

Most proteins, especially milk

TYROSINE (needed by the thyroid)

Most proteins, particularly casein—a milk protein

OXYGEN (in addition to breathing) (needed particularly by the brain)

Horseradish	Potatoes
Mint	Radishes
Onions	Tomatoes
Parsley	

UNSATURATED FATTY ACIDS (see Chapters 6, 13)

Brains	Olive oil
Egg-yolk	Sunflower-seed oil
Lard	Wheat-germ oil
Linseed oil	

APPENDIX D

FOODS THAT CONTAIN ELEMENTS
NECESSARY FOR FEEDING THE BRAIN
See also Chapter 13

"Brain" vitamins

Vitamins E (and D), B complex, particularly B_1, riboflavin, and B_6. See Appendix A for a list of foods that contain these vitamins.

Apples
Apricots
Asparagus
Beef
Black molasses
Brains
Brussels sprouts
Carrots
Cauliflower
Celery
Cherries
Coconut
Cod-liver oil
Cucumber
Currants
Dried fruits
Endives
Egg-yolk (raw)
Figs
Fish
Garlic
Gooseberries
Grapes
Greens

Horseradish
Kidneys
Lard
Lettuce
Liver
Loganberries
Milk
Mint
Mushrooms
Mustard and cress
Nasturtium flowers (in
    salads)
Olive oil
Olives
Onions
Oranges
Oysters
Peas
Potatoes
Pumpkin
Parsley
Radishes
Raspberries
Seafood

Soya beans
Strawberries
Sunflower-seed oil
Turnip-tops
Watercress

Wheat germ
Wheat-germ oil
Whole-meal bread and
  flour
Yellow-stone fruit

APPENDIX E

FOODS THAT CONTAIN ELEMENTS
GLANDS NEED
See also Chapter 5

For the adrenal glands

Vitamins A, C, and E (see Appendix A); tyrosine (see Appendix C)

Plenty of cheese, eggs, fish, meat, milk.

For the gonads (sex glands)

Vitamins A, B, C, E (see Appendix A); arginine (see Appendix C); iron and copper (see Appendix B)

Plenty of meat, eggs, fish, cheese; oatmeal, peanut flour, whole-wheat flour, bread, and wheat germ; lentils, whole barley; liver; kidney beans, parsley, black molasses, mushrooms, asparagus.

For the pituitary gland

Water; Vitamins B and E (see Appendix A); manganese (see Appendix B)

Potatoes, lettuce, wheat germ, walnuts, almonds, liver, peanuts, agar-agar, raw egg-yolk, parsley, olives; plenty of meat, eggs, fish, cheese, milk.

For the parathyroid glands

Vitamin D (see Appendix A); calcium (see Appendix B)

Oranges, apples, cabbage, cucumber, lettuce, radishes, watercress, whole wheat, carrots, beetroot, honey.

For the pancreas

> Vitamin B complex (see Appendix A); sulphur and nickel (see Appendix B); cystine and glutamic acid (see Appendix C)

> Plenty of eggs, milk, meat, fish, cheese; Brussels sprouts, cauliflower, cabbage, lettuce, strawberries, gooseberries, egg-yolk, turnips, onions, coconut, carrots.

For the thymus gland

> Vitamin B complex (see Appendix A)

For the thyroid gland

> Iodine (see Appendix B); Vitamin B and Vitamin C (see Appendix A); tyrosine (see Appendix C)

> All seafood, particularly oysters, shrimps, and salmon; cod-liver oil, all sea-greens; tomatoes, radishes, dark berries, beetroot, asparagus.

APPENDIX F

PLANNING YOUR MENUS
See also Chapter 4

From these lists of foods menus for your three meals daily can easily be chosen. Each meal must be balanced—it must contain protein, carbohydrate, fat, and cleansing and protective elements (fruit, fresh, and green vegetables).

Examples

BREAKFAST

Wheat germ with dried skimmed milk, fresh milk and honey; and/or egg cooked in any way except by frying; or kidneys, grilled bacon, or fish; whole-meal bread, butter, and fresh fruit.

MIDDAY MEAL

Fruit or tomato juice or clear soup; fish, meat, cheese, or egg (if not eaten at breakfast); salad (dressed with wheat-germ or sunflower-seed oil, cider vinegar, or fresh lemon juice), biochemic salt; fresh fruit; yoghurt.

EVENING MEAL

Fruit or tomato juice or clear soup. Meat, fish, cheese, or egg (if not eaten at midday); potatoes in skin, with butter; green vegetables, a root vegetable; fruit jelly made with dried seaweed, kelp, agar-agar; fresh fruit; yoghurt.

(A cooked meal can be eaten at midday and a salad meal in the evening if this is more convenient.)

BEDTIME

Two teaspoonsful of black molasses with milk.

Four tablespoonsful of brewers' yeast should be taken daily in soup, tomato juice, or any other liquid.

APPENDIX G

THE NUTRITIVE VALUE OF FOODS

NUTRITIVE VALUE
OF FOODS

Courtesy of Institute of Home Economics
Agriculture Research Service

APPENDIX G

NUTRITIVE VALUE OF FOODS

A glass of milk . . . a slice of cooked meat . . . an apple . . . a slice of bread—what food values does each contain? How much cooked meat will a pound of raw meat yield?

Ready answers to questions like these are helpful to homemakers who need quantitative information for the planning of nutritionally adequate diets, and to nutritionists, dieticians, and physicians.

The answers will be found in the two tables provided in the following pages.

EXPLANATION OF THE TABLES

ABOUT TABLE 1

Table 1 shows the food values in about 500 foods commonly used in this country.

Foods listed.—Foods are grouped under the following main headings: Milk; eggs; meat, poultry, and fish; dry beans and peas, nuts; vegetables; fruits; grain products; fats; sugars; and miscellaneous items.

Most of the foods listed are in ready-to-eat form. Some are basic products widely used in food preparation, such as flour, fat, and cornmeal.

Weight in grams is shown for an approximate measure of each food as it is described; if inedible parts are included in the description, both measure and weight include these parts.

The approximate measure shown for each food is in cups, ounces, pounds, a piece of a certain size, or some other well-known unit. The measure shown can be calculated readily to larger or smaller amounts by multiplying or dividing. However, because the measures are approximate (some are rounded for convenient use), calculated

221

nutritive values for very large quantities of some food items may be less representative than those for smaller quantities.

The cup measure refers to the standard measuring cup of 8 fluid ounces or ½ liquid pint. The ounce refers to ¹⁄₁₆ of a pound avoirdupois, unless fluid ounce is indicated. The weight of a fluid ounce varies according to the food measured.

Shown below are the equivalents for most of the measures used in the food listings.

EQUIVALENTS BY WEIGHT

1 pound (16 ounces)	= 453.6 grams
1 ounce	= 28.35 grams
3½ ounces	= 100 grams

EQUIVALENTS BY VOLUME

(All measurements level)

1 quart	= 4 cups
1 cup	= 8 fluid ounces
	= ½ pint
	= 16 tablespoons
2 tablespoons	= 1 fluid ounce
1 tablespoon	= 3 teaspoons
1 pound butter or margarine	= 4 sticks
	= 2 cups
	= 64 pats or squares
1 stick butter or margarine	= ½ cup (approximately)
	= 16 pats or squares

Food values.—Values are shown for protein; fat; fatty acids; total carbohydrate; two minerals—calcium and iron; and five vitamins—vitamin A, thiamine, riboflavin, niacin, and ascorbic acid (vitamin C). Calories are shown also, in the column headed "Food energy." The calorie is the unit of measure for the energy furnished the body by protein, fat, and carbohydrate.

These values can be used as the basis for comparing kinds and amounts of nutrients in different foods. For some foods, the values can be used in comparing different forms of the same food.

Water content is also shown in the table because the percentage of moisture present is needed for identification and comparison of many food items.

Nutritive values are shown for only the parts of food customarily eaten—corn without the cob, meat without bone, potatoes without the skin, American-type grapes without seeds and skin, European-type grapes without seeds. If additional parts are eaten—the skin of the potato, for example—amounts of some nutrients obtained will be somewhat greater than those shown.

For many of the prepared items, values have been calculated from the ingredients in typical recipes. Examples of such items are: Biscuits, corn muffins, oyster stew, macaroni and cheese, and custard and a number of other dessert-type items.

For vegetables and for toast, the values are shown for the food without any fat added, either during preparation or at the table.

For meat, the values are for the meat as cooked and drained and without drippings. For many cuts, values are shown for the meat both with and without the fat that can be trimmed off in the kitchen or on the plate.

ABOUT TABLE 2

Meat undergoes certain losses from the time it is purchased to the time it is ready to serve. Among these losses are those that occur through evaporation of moisture, loss of fat in the drippings, and discard of bone and various trimmings.

Table 2 can be used as a guide to the amount of raw meat to buy in order to have a given amount of cooked meat to serve.

It shows the approximate weight of cooked, drained meat that usually can be expected from a pound of raw meat as purchased in several familiar cuts. Yield is given as ounces of—

Cooked meat with bone and fat
Cooked meat without bone, with fat
Cooked lean and fat
Cooked lean only

Among the factors that influence the yield of meat is the proportion of fat and lean in the piece. Many cuts have a layer of fat extending all or part way around. The thickness of this fat varies because practices in cutting and trimming meat to retail bases differ widely. The data in table 2, as well as those in table 1, apply to cuts trimmed so that the outer layer of fat is not more than 1/2 inch in width. Deposits of fat within a cut may be extensive; these usually are not affected by retail trimming though they may be discarded at the table.

TABLES I and II

THE NUTRITIVE VALUE OF FOODS

APPENDIX G

	Food, approximate measure, and weight (in grams)			Water	Food energy	Protein	Fat (total lipid)
	MILK, CREAM, CHEESE; RELATED PRODUCTS						
	Milk, cow's:		Grams	Per-cent	Calo-ries	Grams	Grams
1	Fluid, whole_____	1 cup_____	244__	87	165	9	10
2	Fluid, nonfat (skim)_____	1 cup_____	246__	90	90	9	Trace
3	Buttermilk, cultured, from skim milk.	1 cup_____	246__	90	90	9	Trace
4	Evaporated, unsweetened, undiluted.	1 cup_____	252__	74	345	18	20
5	Condensed, sweetened, un-diluted.	1 cup_____	306__	26	985	25	25
6	Dry, whole_____	1 cup_____	103__	2	515	27	28
7	Dry, nonfat_____	1 cup_____	80___	3	290	29	1
8	Milk, goat's: Fluid, whole____	1 cup_____	244__	88	165	8	10
	Cream:						
9	Half-and-half (milk and cream).	1 cup_____	242__	80	330	8	29
10		1 tablespoon__	15___	80	20	Trace	2
11	Light, table or coffee_____	1 cup_____	240__	71	525	7	52
12		1 tablespoon__	15___	71	35	Trace	3
	Whipping, unwhipped (volume about double when whipped):						
13	Medium_____	1 cup_____	239__	61	745	6	78
14		1 tablespoon__	15___	61	45	Trace	5
15	Heavy_____	1 cup_____	238__	56	860	5	93
16		1 tablespoon__	15___	56	55	Trace	6
	Cheese:						
17	Blue mold (Roquefort type)_	1 ounce_____	28___	40	105	6	9
	Cheddar or American:						
18	Ungrated_____	1-inch cube___	17___	36	70	4	6
19	Grated_____	1 cup_____	112__	36	455	28	37
20		1 tablespoon__	7____	36	30	2	2
21	Cheddar, process_____	1 ounce_____	28___	39	105	7	9
22	Cheese foods, Cheddar_____	1 ounce_____	28___	43	95	6	7

| Fatty acids | | | Carbo-hy-drate | Cal-cium | Iron | Vita-min A value | Thia-mine | Ribo-flavin | Nia-cin | Ascor-bic acid |
| Satu-rated (total) | Unsaturated | | | | | | | | | |
	Oleic	Lino-leic								
Grams	Grams	Grams	Grams	Milli-grams	Milli-grams	Inter-national Units	Milli-grams	Milli-grams	Milli-grams	Milli-grams
6	3	Trace	12	285	0.1	390	0.08	0.42	0.2	2
-----	-----	-----	13	298	.1	10	.10	.44	.2	2
-----	-----	-----	13	298	.1	10	.10	.44	.2	2
11	7	1	24	635	.3	820	.10	.84	.5	3
14	8	1	170	829	.3	1,020	.24	1.21	.5	3
15	9	1	39	968	.5	1,160	.30	1.50	.7	6
-----	-----	-----	42	1,040	.5	20	.28	1.44	.7	6
6	2	Trace	11	315	.2	390	.10	.27	.7	2
16	10	1	11	259	.1	1,190	.07	.39	.1	2
1	1	Trace	1	16	0	70	0	.02	0	Trace
29	17	2	10	238	.1	2,140	.07	.35	.1	Trace
2	1	Trace	1	15	0	130	0	.02	0	Trace
43	26	2	8	196	.1	3,200	.06	.29	.1	Trace
3	2	Trace	1	12	0	200	0	.02	0	Trace
51	31	3	7	164	0	3,800	.05	.24	.1	Trace
3	2	Trace	Trace	10	0	240	0	.02	0	Trace
5	3	Trace	Trace	122	.2	350	.01	.17	.1	0
3	2	Trace	Trace	133	.2	230	Trace	.08	Trace	0
20	12	1	2	874	1.2	1,510	.03	.53	.1	0
1	1	Trace	Trace	55	.1	90	.02	.03	Trace	0
5	3	Trace	Trace	214	.2	350	Trace	.12	Trace	0
4	2	Trace	2	163	.2	300	.01	.17	Trace	0

Food, approximate measure, and weight (in grams)			Water	Food energy	Protein	Fat (total lipid)

MILK, CREAM, CHEESE—Continued

				Per-cent	Calo-ries	Grams	Grams
	Cheese—Continued						
	Cottage cheese, from skim milk:		Grams				
23	Creamed_____	1 cup_____	225__	78	240	30	11
24		1 ounce_____	28___	78	30	4	1
25	Uncreamed_____	1 cup_____	225__	79	195	38	1
26		1 ounce_____	28___	79	25	5	Trace
27	Cream cheese_____	1 ounce_____	28___	51	105	2	11
28		1 tablespoon__	15___	51	55	1	6
29	Swiss_____	1 ounce_____	28___	39	105	7	8
	Milk beverages:						
30	Cocoa_____	1 cup_____	242__	79	235	9	11
31	Chocolate-flavored milk drink.	1 cup_____	250__	83	190	8	6
32	Malted milk_____	1 cup_____	270__	78	280	13	12
	Milk desserts:						
33	Cornstarch pudding, plain (blanc mange).	1 cup_____	248__	76	275	9	10
34	Custard, baked_____	1 cup_____	248__	77	285	13	14
	Ice cream, plain, factory packed:						
35	Slice or cut brick, ⅛ of quart brick.	1 slice or cut brick.	71___	62	145	3	9
36	Container_____	3½ fluid ounces.	62___	62	130	2	8
37	Container_____	8 fluid ounces_	142__	62	295	6	18
38	Ice milk_____	1 cup_____	187__	67	285	9	10
39	Yoghurt, from partially skimmed milk.	1 cup_____	246__	89	120	8	4

EGGS

	Eggs, large, 24 ounces per dozen:						
	Raw:						
40	Whole, without shell_____	1 egg_____	50___	74	80	6	6

| Fatty acids | | | Carbo-hy-drate | Cal-cium | Iron | Vita-min A value | Thia-mine | Ribo-flavin | Nia-cin | Ascor-bic acid |
| Satu-rated (total) | Unsaturated | | | | | | | | | |
	Oleic	Lino-leic								
Grams	Grams	Grams	Grams	Milli-grams	Milli-grams	Inter-national Units	Milli-grams	Milli-grams	Milli-grams	Milli-grams
6	4	Trace	6	207	0.9	430	0.07	0.66	0.2	0
1	Trace	Trace	1	25	.1	50	.01	.08	Trace	0
Trace	Trace	Trace	6	202	.9	20	.07	.64	.2	0
-----	-----	-----	1	26	.1	Trace	.01	.08	Trace	0
6	4	Trace	1	18	.1	440	Trace	.07	Trace	0
3	2	Trace	Trace	9	Trace	230	Trace	.04	Trace	0
4	3	Trace	1	271	.3	320	.01	.06	Trace	0
6	4	Trace	26	286	.9	390	.09	.45	.4	2
3	2	Trace	27	270	.4	210	.09	.41	.2	2
7	4	Trace	32	364	.8	670	.17	.56	-----	2
6	3	Trace	39	290	.1	390	.07	.40	.1	2
6	5	1	28	278	1.0	870	.10	.47	.2	1
5	3	Trace	15	87	.1	370	.03	.13	.1	1
4	3	Trace	13	76	.1	320	.03	.12	.1	1
10	6	1	29	175	.1	740	.06	.27	.1	1
6	3	Trace	42	292	.2	390	.09	.41	.2	2
2	1	Trace	13	295	.1	170	.09	.43	.2	2
2	3	Trace	Trace	27	1.1	590	.05	.15	Trace	0

41	White of egg_____	1 white_____	33___	88	15	4	Trace
42	Yolk of egg_____	1 yolk_____	17___	51	60	3	5
	Cooked:						
43	Boiled, shell removed____	2 eggs_____	100__	74	160	13	12
44	Scrambled, with milk and fat.	1 egg_____	64___	72	110	7	8

MEAT, POULTRY, FISH, SHELLFISH; RELATED PRODUCTS

45	Bacon, broiled or fried crisp__	2 slices_____	16___	8	95	5	8
	Beef, trimmed to retail basis,[1] cooked:						
	Cuts braised, simmered, or pot-roasted:						
46	Lean and fat_____	3 ounces_____	85___	53	245	23	16
47	Lean only_____	2.5 ounces____	72___	62	140	22	5
	Hamburger, broiled:						
48	Market ground_____	3 ounces_____	85___	54	245	21	17
49	Ground lean_____	3 ounces_____	85___	60	185	23	10
	Roast, oven-cooked, no liquid added:						
	Relatively fat, such as rib:						
50	Lean and fat_____	3 ounces_____	85___	38	390	16	36
51	Lean only_____	1.8 ounces____	51___	57	120	14	7
	Relatively lean, such as round:						
52	Lean and fat_____	3 ounces_____	85___	56	220	23	14
53	Lean only_____	2.5 ounces_____	71___	63	130	21	4
	Steak, broiled:						
	Relatively fat, such as sirloin:						
54	Lean and fat_____	3 ounces_____	85___	44	330	20	27
55	Lean only_____	2 ounces_____	56___	59	115	18	4
	Relatively lean, such as round:						
56	Lean and fat_____	3 ounces_____	85___	55	220	24	13
57	Lean only_____	2.4 ounces____	69___	61	130	22	
	Beef, canned:						
58	Corned beef_____	3 ounces_____	85___	59	180	22	10
59	Corned beef hash_____	3 ounces_____	85___	70	120	12	5
60	Beef, dried or chipped_____	2 ounces_____	57___	48	115	19	4
61	Beef and vegetable stew_____	1 cup_____	235__	82	185	15	10
62	Beef potpie, baked: Individual pie, 4¼-inch-diameter, weight before baking about 8 ounces.	1 pie_____	227__	63	460	18	28
	Chicken, cooked:						
63	Flesh and skin, broiled_____	3 ounces without bone.	85___	61	185	23	9

[1] Outer layer of fat on the cut was removed to within approximately ½ inch

			Trace	3	Trace	0	Trace	.09	Trace	0
2	2	Trace	Trace	24	.9	580	.04	.07	Trace	0
	5	1	1	54	2.3	1,180	.09	.28	.1	0
3	4	1	1	51	1.1	690	.05	.18	Trace	0
3	4	1	1	2	.5	0	.08	.05	.8	------
8	7	Trace	0	10	2.9	30	.04	.18	3.5	------
2	2	Trace	0	10	2.7	10	.04	.16	3.3	------
8	7	Trace	0	9	2.7	30	.07	.02	4.6	------
5	4	Trace	0	10	3.0	20	.08	.20	5.1	------
17	16	1	0	7	2.1	70	.04	.13	3.0	------
3	3	Trace	0	6	1.8	10	.04	.11	2.6	------
7	6	Trace	0	10	3.0	30	.06	.18	4.2	------
2	2	Trace	0	9	2.7	10	.05	.16	3.8	------
13	12	1	0	8	2.5	50	.05	.16	4.0	------
2	2	Trace	0	7	2.2	10	.05	.14	3.6	------
6	6	Trace	0	11	3.0	20	.07	.19	4.8	------
2	2	Trace	0	9	2.6	10	.06	.16	4.2	------
5	4	Trace	0	17	3.7	20	.01	.20	2.9	------
2	2	Trace	6	22	1.1	10	.02	.11	2.4	------
2	2	Trace	0	11	2.9	------	.04	.18	2.2	------
.5	4	Trace	15	31	2.8	2,530	.13	.18	4.4	14
10	15	1	32	20	2.5	2,830	.07	.14	3.0	Trace
3	4	2	0	10	1.4	260	.04	.15	7.1	------

of the lean. Deposits of fat within the cut were not removed.

Food, approximate measure, and weight (in grams)			Water	Food energy	Protein	Fat (total lipid)

MEAT, POULTRY, FISH, SHELLFISH—Continued

				Per- cent	Calo- ries	Grams	Grams
	Chicken, cooked—Continued		Grams				
	Breast, fried, ½ breast:						
64	With bone_____	3.3 ounces____	94___	52	215	24	12
65	Flesh and skin only_____	2.8 ounces____	79___	52	215	24	12
	Leg, fried (thigh and drumstick):						
66	With bone_____	4.3 ounces____	121__	52	245	27	15
67	Flesh and skin only_____	3.1 ounces____	89___	52	245	27	15
68	Chicken, canned, boneless____	3 ounces_____	85___	62	170	25·	7
	Chicken potpie. See Poultry potpie.						
	Chile con carne, canned:						
69	With beans_____	1 cup_____	250__	72	335	19	15
70	Without beans_____	1 cup_____	255__	67	510	26	38
71	Heart, beef, trimmed of fat, braised.	3 ounces_____	85___	61	160	26	5
	Lamb, trimmed to retail basis,[1] cooked:						
72	Chop, thick, with bone, broiled.	1 chop, 4.8 ounces.	137__	47	405	25	33
73	Lean and fat_____	4 ounces_____	112__	47	405	25	33
74	Lean only _____	2.6 ounces____	74___	62	140	21	6
	Leg, roasted:						
75	Lean and fat_____	3 ounces_____	85___	54	235	22	16
76	Lean only_____	2.5 ounces____	71___	62	130	20	5
	Shoulder, roasted:						
77	Lean and fat_____	3 ounces_____	85___	50	285	18	23
78	Lean only_____	2.3 ounces____	64___	61	130	17	6
79	Liver, beef, fried_____	2 ounces_____	57___	57	120	13	4
	Pork, cured, cooked:						
80	Ham, smoked, lean and fat_	3 ounces_____	85___	48	290	18	24
	Luncheon meat:						
81	Cooked ham, sliced_____	2 ounces_____	57___	48	170	13	13
82	Canned, spiced or unspiced_	2 ounces_____	57___	55	165	8	14

Fatty acids			Carbo-hy-drate	Cal-cium	Iron	Vita-min A value	Thia-mine	Ribo-flavin	Nia-cin	Ascor-bic acid
Satu-rated (total)	Unsaturated									
	Oleic	Lino-leic								
Grams	Grams	Grams	Grams	Milli-grams	Milli-grams	Inter-national Units	Milli-grams	Milli-grams	Milli-grams	Milli-grams
3	6	2	------	10	1.1	60	0.03	0.06	9.4	------
3	6	2	------	10	1.1	60	.03	.06	9.4	------
4	7	2	------	13	1.8	220	.05	.18	4.7	------
4	7	2	------	13	1.8	220	.05	.18	4.7	------
2	3	1	0	12	1.5	160	.03	.14	5.4	------
7	7	Trace	30	98	4.2	150	.08	.20	3.5	------
18	17	1	15	97	3.6	380	.05	.31	5.6	------
2	2	Trace	1	14	5.9	30	.23	1.05	6.8	3
18	12	1	0	10	3.1	--------	.14	.25	4.5	------
18	12	1	0	10	3.1	--------	.14	.25	5.6	------
3	2	Trace	0	9	2.5	--------	.11	.20	4.5	------
9	6	Trace	0	9	2.8	--------	.13	.23	4.7	------
3	2	Trace	0	9	2.6	--------	.12	.21	4.4	------
13	8	1	0	8	2.4	--------	.11	.20	4.0	------
3	2	Trace	0	8	2.2	--------	.10	.18	3.7	------
2	2	Trace	6	5	4.4	30,330	.15	2.25	8.4	18
9	10	2	1	8	2.2	0	.39	.15	3.1	------
5	5	1	0	5	1.5	0	.57	.15	2.9	------
5	6	1	1	5	1.2	0	.18	.12	1.6	------

	Pork, fresh, trimmed to retail basis,[1] cooked:						
83	Chop, thick, with bone____	1 chop, 3.5 ounces.	98___	42	260	16	21
84	Lean and fat____	2.3 ounces____	66___	42	260	16	21
85	Lean only____	1.7 ounces____	48___	53	130	15	7
	Roast, oven-cooked, no liquid added:						
86	Lean and fat____	3 ounces____	85___	46	310	21	24
87	Lean only____	2.4 ounces____	68___	55	175	20	10
	Cuts simmered:						
88	Lean and fat____	3 ounces____	85___	46	320	20	26
89	Lean only____	2.2 ounces____	63___	60	135	18	6
90	Poultry potpie (chicken or turkey): Individual pie, 4¼-inch-diameter, about 8 ounces.	1 pie____	227__	60	485	17	28
	Sausage:						
91	Bologna, slice 4.1 by 0.1 inch.	8 slices____	227__	56	690	27	62
92	Frankfurter, cooked____	1 frankfurter__	51___	58	155	6	14
93	Pork, bulk, canned____	4 ounces____	113__	55	340	18	29
94	Tongue, beef, simmered____	3 ounces____	85___	61	205	18	14
	Turkey potpie. *See* Poultry potpie.						
	Veal, cooked:						
95	Cutlet, broiled____	3 ounces without bone.	85___	60	185	23	9
96	Roast, medium fat, medium done: Lean and fat.	3 ounces____	85___	55	305	23	14
	Fish and shellfish:						
97	Bluefish, baked or broiled_	3 ounces____	85___	68	135	22	4
	Clams:						
98	Raw, meat only____	3 ounces____	85___	80	70	11	1
99	Canned, solids and liquid_	3 ounces____	85___	87	45	7	1
100	Crabmeat, canned or cooked.	3 ounces____	85___	77	90	14	2
101	Fishsticks, breaded, cooked, frozen; stick, 3.8 by 1.0 by 0.5 inch.	10 sticks or 8-ounce package.	227__	66	400	38	20
102	Haddock, fried____	3 ounces____	85___	67	135	16	5
	Mackerel:						
103	Broiled, Atlantic____	3 ounces____	85___	62	200	19	13
104	Canned, Pacific, solids and liquid.	3 ounces____	85___	66	155	18	9

[1] Outer layer of fat on the cut was removed to within approximately ½ inch

8	9	2	0	8	2.2	0	.63	.18	3.8	------
8	9	2	0	8	2.2	0	.63	.18	3.8	------
3	3	1	0	7	1.9	0	.54	.16	3.3	------
9	10	2	0	9	2.7	0	.78	.22	4.7	------
4	4	1	0	9	2.6	0	.73	.21	4.4	------
9	11	2	0	8	2.5	0	.46	.21	4.1	------
2	3	1	0	8	2.3	0	.42	.19	3.7	------
8	15	3	39	41	1.6	1,860	.07	.14	3.2	Trace
26	27	3	2	16	4.1	--------	.36	.49	6.0	------
6	6	1	1	3	.8	--------	.08	.10	1.3	------
10	12	3	0	10	2.6	0	.23	.27	3.4	------
7	6	Trace	Trace	7	2.5	--------	.04	.26	3.1	------
4	4	Trace	0	9	2.7	--------	.06	.21	4.6	------
7	6	Trace	0	10	2.9	--------	.11	.26	6.6	------
------	------	------	0	25	.6	40	.09	.08	1.6	------
------	------	------	3	82	6.0	90	.08	.15	1.4	------
------	------	------	2	74	5.4	70	.04	.08	.9	------
------	------	------	1	38	.8	--------	.04	.05	2.1	------
5	4	10	15	25	.9	--------	.09	.16	3.6	------
1	3	Trace	6	15	.5	50	.03	.08	2.2	------
------	------	------	0	5	1.0	450	.13	.23	6.5	------
------	------	------	0	221	1.9	20	.02	.28	7.4	------

of the lean. Deposits of fat within the cut were not removed.

Food, approximate measure, and weight (in grams)			Water	Food energy	Protein	Fat (total lipid)
			Percent	*Calories*	*Grams*	*Grams*

MEAT, POULTRY, FISH, SHELLFISH—Continued

	Fish and shellfish—Continued		*Grams*	*Percent*	*Calories*	*Grams*	*Grams*
105	Ocean perch, breaded (egg and breadcrumbs), fried.	3 ounces_____	85___	59	195	16	11
106	Oysters, meat only: Raw, 13–19 medium selects.	1 cup_____	240__	85	160	20	4
107	Oyster stew, 1 part oysters to 3 parts milk by volume, 3–4 oysters.	1 cup_____	230__	84	200	11	12
108	Salmon, pink, canned_____	3 ounces_____	85___	70	120	17	5
109	Sardines, Atlantic type, canned in oil, drained solids.	3 ounces_____	85___	57	180	22	9
110	Shad, baked_____	3 ounces_____	85___	64	170	20	10
111	Shrimp, canned, meat only_	3 ounces_____	85___	66	110	23	1
112	Swordfish, broiled with butter or margarine.	3 ounces_____	85___	65	150	24	5
113	Tuna, canned in oil, drained solids.	3 ounces_____	85___	60	170	25	7

MATURE DRY BEANS AND PEAS, NUTS, PEANUTS; RELATED PRODUCTS

114	Almonds, shelled_____	1 cup_____	142__	5	850	26	77
	Beans, dry:						
	Common varieties, such as Great Northern, navy, and others, canned:						
115	Red_____	1 cup_____	256__	76	230	15	1
	White, with tomato or molasses:						
116	With pork_____	1 cup_____	261__	69	330	16	7
117	Without pork_____	1 cup_____	261__	69	315	16	1
118	Lima, cooked_____	1 cup_____	192__	64	260	16	1

Fatty acids			Carbo-hy-drate	Cal-cium	Iron	Vita-min A value	Thia-mine	Ribo-flavin	Nia-cin	Ascor-bic acid
Satu-rated (total)	Unsaturated									
	Oleic	Lino-leic								
Grams	Grams	Grams	Grams	Milli-grams	Milli-grams	Inter-national Units	Milli-grams	Milli-grams	Milli-grams	Milli-grams
------	------	------	6	14	1.3	50	0.09	0.10	1.7	------
------	------	------	8	226	13.2	740	.30	.39	6.6	------
------	------	------	11	269	3.3	640	.12	.40	1.7	------
1	1	------	0	2 159	.7	60	.03	.16	6.8	------
2	2	4	1	367	2.5	190	.02	.18	4.6	------
------	------	------	0	20	.5	20	.11	.22	7.3	------
------	------	------		98	2.6	50	.01	.03	1.9	------
------	------	------	0	23	1.1	1,750	.03	.04	9.3	------
2	1	4	0	7	1.2	70	.04	.10	10.9	------
6	52	15	28	332	6.7	0	.34	1.31	5.0	Trace
------	------	------	42	74	4.6	0	.13	.13	1.5	Trace
3	3	1	54	172	4.4	140	.13	.10	1.3	5
------	------	------	60	183	5.2	140	.13	.10	1.3	5
------	------	------	48	56	5.6	Trace	.26	.12	1.3	Trace

119	Brazil nuts, broken pieces	1 cup	140	5	905	20	92
120	Cashew nuts, roasted	1 cup	135	5	770	25	65
	Coconut:						
121	Fresh, shredded	1 cup	97	50	330	3	31
122	Dried, shredded, sweetened	1 cup	62	3	345	2	24
123	Cowpeas or blackeye peas, dry, cooked.	1 cup	248	80	190	13	1
	Peanuts, roasted, shelled:						
124	Halves	1 cup	144	2	840	39	71
125	Chopped	1 tablespoon	9	2	50	2	4
126	Peanut butter	1 tablespoon	16	2	90	4	8
127	Peas, split, dry, cooked	1 cup	250	70	290	20	1
	Pecans:						
128	Halves	1 cup	108	3	740	10	77
129	Chopped	1 tablespoon	7.5	3	50	1	5
	Walnuts, shelled:						
130	Black or native, chopped	1 cup	126	3	790	26	75
	English or Persian:						
131	Halves	1 cup	100	4	650	15	64
132	Chopped	1 tablespoon	8	4	50	1	5

VEGETABLES AND VEGETABLE PRODUCTS

	Asparagus:						
133	Cooked, cut spears	1 cup	175	92	35	4	Trace
	Canned spears, medium:						
134	Green	6 spears	96	92	20	2	Trace
135	Bleached	6 spears	96	92	20	2	Trace
	Beans:						
136	Lima, immature, cooked	1 cup	160	75	150	8	1
	Snap, green: Cooked:						
137	In small amount of water, short time.	1 cup	125	92	25	2	Trace
138	In large amount of water, long time.	1 cup	125	92	25	2	Trace
	Canned:						
139	Solids and liquid	1 cup	239	94	45	2	Trace
140	Strained or chopped	1 ounce	28	93	5	Trace	Trace
	Bean sprouts. See Sprouts.						
141	Beets, cooked, diced	1 cup	165	88	70	2	Trace
142	Broccoli spears, cooked	1 cup	150	90	45	5	Trace
143	Brussels sprouts, cooked	1 cup	130	85	60	6	1

2 If bones are discarded, calcium content is much lower. Bones equal about

18	44	24	15	260	4.8	Trace	1.21	------	------	------
11	46	5	35	51	5.1	--------	.49	.46	1.9	------
27	2	------	13	15	1.7	0	.06	.03	.5	4
21	2	------	33	13	1.6	0	.04	.02	.4	0
------	------	------	34	42	3.2	20	.41	.11	1.1	Trace
16	31	21	28	104	3.2	0	.47	.19	24.6	0
1	2	1	2	6	.2	0	.03	.01	1.5	0
2	4	2	3	12	.4	0	.02	.02	2.8	0
------	------	------	52	28	4.2	120	.36	.22	2.2	Trace
5	49	15	16	79	2.6	140	.93	.14	1.0	2
Trace	3	1	1	5	.2	10	.06	.01	.1	Trace
4	26	36	19	Trace	7.6	380	.28	.14	.9	------
4	10	40	16	99	3.1	30	.33	.13	.9	3
Trace	1	3	1	8	.2	Trace	.03	.01	.1	Trace
------	------	------	6	33	1.8	1,820	.23	.30	2.1	40
------	------	------	3	18	1.8	770	.06	.08	.9	17
------	------	------	4	15	1.0	70	.05	.07	.8	17
------	------	------	29	46	2.7	460	.22	.14	1.8	24
------	------	------	6	45	.9	830	.09	.12	.6	18
------	------	------	6	45	.9	830	.06	.11	.5	12
------	------	------	10	65	3.3	990	.08	.10	.7	9
------	------	------	1	10	.3	120	.01	.02	.1	1
------	------	------	16	35	1.2	30	.03	.07	.5	11
------	------	------	8	195	2.0	5,100	.10	.22	1.2	111
------	------	------	12	44	1.7	520	.05	.16	.6	61

2 percent by weight of total contents of can.

Food, approximate measure, and weight (in grams)			Water	Food energy	Protein	Fat (total lipid)

VEGETABLES—Continued

	Cabbage:		Grams	Percent	Calories	Grams	Grams
	Raw:						
144	Finely shredded	1 cup	100	92	25	1	Trace
145	Coleslaw	1 cup	120	84	100	2	7
	Cooked:						
146	In small amount of water, short time.	1 cup	170	92	40	2	Trace
147	In large amount of water, long time.	1 cup	170	92	40	2	Trace
	Cabbage, celery or Chinese:						
148	Raw, leaves and stem, 1-inch pieces.	1 cup	100	95	15	1	Trace
149	Cooked	1 cup	190	95	25	2	1
	Carrots:						
	Raw:						
150	Whole, 5½ by 1 inch (25 thin strips).	1 carrot	50	88	20	1	Trace
151	Grated	1 cup	110	88	45	1	Trace
152	Cooked, diced	1 cup	145	92	45	1	1
153	Canned, strained or chopped.	1 ounce	28	92	.5	Trace	0
154	Cauliflower, cooked, flower-buds.	1 cup	120	92	30	3	Trace
	Celery, raw:						
155	Stalk, large outer, 8 by about 1½ inches at root end.	1 stalk	40	94	5	1	Trace
156	Pieces, diced	1 cup	100	94	20	1	Trace
157	Collards, cooked	1 cup	190	87	75	7	1
	Corn, sweet:						
158	Cooked, ear 5 by 1¾ inches.	1 ear	140	76	65	2	1
159	Canned, solids and liquid	1 cup	256	80	170	5	1
160	Cowpeas, cooked, immature seeds.	1 cup	160	75	150	11	1

Fatty acids			Carbo-hy-drate	Cal-cium	Iron	Vita-min A value	Thia-mine	Ribo-flavin	Nia-cin	Ascor-bic acid
Satu-rated (total)	Unsaturated									
	Oleic	Lino-leic								
Grams	Grams	Grams	Grams	Milli-grams	Milli-grams	Inter-national Units	Milli-grams	Milli-grams	Milli-grams	Milli-grams
-----	-----	-----	5	46	0.5	80	0.06	0.05	0.3	50
1	1	4	9	47	.5	80	.06	.05	.3	50
-----	-----	-----	9	78	.8	150	.08	.08	.5	53
-----	-----	-----	9	78	.8	150	.05	.05	.3	32
-----	-----	-----	2	43	.9	260	.03	.04	.4	31
-----	-----	-----	5	82	1.7	490	.04	.06	.6	42
-----	-----	-----	5	20	.4	6,000	.03	.03	.3	3
-----	-----	-----	10	43	.9	13,200	.06	.06	.7	7
-----	-----	-----	9	38	.9	18,130	.07	.07	.7	6
-----	-----	-----	2	7	.2	3,400	.01	.01	.1	1
-----	-----	-----	6	26	1.3	110	.07	.10	.6	34
-----	-----	-----	1	20	.2	0	.02	.02	.2	3
-----	-----	-----	4	50	.5	0	.05	.04	.4	7
-----	-----	-----	14	473	3.0	14,500	.15	.46	3.2	84
-----	-----	-----	16	4	.5	[3] 300	.09	.08	1.1	6
-----	-----	-----	41	10	1.3	[3] 520	.07	.13	2.4	14
-----	-----	-----	25	59	4.0	620	.46	.13	1.3	32

	Cucumbers, 10-ounce; 7½ by about 2 inches:						
161	Raw, pared_____	1 cucumber___	207__	96	25	1	Trace
162	Raw, pared, center slice ⅛-inch thick.	6 slices_____	50___	96	5	Trace	Trace
163	Dandelion greens, cooked____	1 cup_____	180__	86	80	5	1
164	Endive, curly (including escarole).	2 ounces_____	57___	93	10	1	Trace
165	Kale, cooked_____	1 cup_____	110__	87	45	4	1
	Lettuce, headed, raw:						
166	Head, looseleaf, 4-inch-diameter.	1 head_____	220__	95	30	3	Trace
167	Head, compact, 4¾-inch-diameter, 1 pound.	1 head_____	454__	95	70	5	1
168	Leaves_____	2 large or 4 small.	50___	95	5	1	Trace
169	Mushrooms, canned, solids and liquid.	1 cup_____	244__	93	30	3	Trace
170	Mustard greens, cooked_____	1 cup_____	140__	92	30	3	Trace
171	Okra, cooked, pod 3 by ⅝ inch.	8 pods_____	85___	90	30	2	Trace
	Onions:						
	Mature:						
172	Raw, onion 2½-inch-diameter.	1 onion_____	110__	88	50	2	Trace
173	Cooked_____	1 cup_____	210__	90	80	2	Trace
174	Young green, small, without tops.	6 onions_____	50___	88	25	Trace	Trace
175	Parsley, raw, chopped_____	1 tablespoon__	3.5__	84	1	Trace	Trace
176	Parsnips, cooked_____	1 cup_____	155__	84	95	2	1
	Peas, green:						
177	Cooked_____	1 cup_____	160__	82	110	8	1
178	Canned, solids and liquid___	1 cup_____	249__	82	170	8	1
179	Canned, strained_____	1 ounce_____	28___	86	10	1	Trace
180	Peppers, hot, red, without seeds, dried; ground chili powder.	1 tablespoon__	15___	13	50	2	1
	Peppers, sweet:						
	Raw, medium, about 6 per pound:						
181	Green pod without stem and seeds.	1 pod_____	62___	93	15	1	Trace
182	Red pod without stem and seeds.	1 pod_____	60___	91	20	1	Trace
183	Canned, pimientos, medium_	1 pod_____	38___	92	10	Trace	Trace
	Potatoes, medium, about 3 per pound:						
184	Baked, peeled after baking_	1 potato_____	99___	75	90	3	Trace

3 Vitamin A value is based on yellow corn; white corn contains only a trace.

-----	-----	-----	6	21	.6	0	.07	.09	.4	18
-----	-----	-----	1	5	.2	0	.02	.02	.1	4
-----	-----	-----	16	337	5.6	27,310	.23	.22	1.3	29
-----	-----	-----	2	45	1.0	1,700	.04	.07	.2	6
-----	-----	-----	8	248	2.4	9,220	.08	.25	1.9	56
-----	-----	-----	6	48	1.1	1,200	.10	.18	.4	17
-----	-----	-----	13	100	2.3	2,470	.20	.38	.9	35
-----	-----	-----	1	11	.2	270	.02	.04	.1	4
-----	-----	-----	9	17	2.0	0	.04	.60	4.8	------
-----	-----	-----	6	308	4.1	10,050	.08	.25	1.0	63
-----	-----	-----	6	70	.6	630	.05	.05	.7	17
-----	-----	-----	11	35	.6	60	.04	.04	.2	10
-----	-----	-----	18	67	1.0	110	.04	.06	.4	13
-----	-----	-----	5	68	.4	30	.02	.02	.1	12
-----	-----	-----	Trace	7	.2	290	Trace	.01	.1	7
-----	-----	-----	22	88	1.1	0	.09	.16	.3	19
-----	-----	-----	19	35	3.0	1,150	.40	.22	3.7	24
-----	-----	-----	32	62	4.5	1,350	.28	.15	2.6	21
-----	-----	-----	2	5	.3	160	.03	.02	.3	2
-----	-----	-----	9	20	1.2	11,520	.03	.20	1.6	2
-----	-----	-----	3	6	.4	260	.05	.05	.3	79
-----	-----	-----	4	8	.4	2,670	.05	.05	.3	122
-----	-----	-----	2	3	.6	870	.01	.02	.1	36
-----	-----	-----	21	9	.7	Trace	.10	.04	1.7	20

Food, approximate measure, and weight (in grams)			Water	Food energy	Protein	Fat (total lipid)

VEGETABLES—Continued

	Food, approximate measure, and weight (in grams)			Per-cent	Calo-ries	Grams	Grams
	Potatoes—Continued						
	Boiled:		Grams				
185	Peeled after boiling	1 potato	136	80	105	3	Trace
186	Peeled before boiling	1 potato	122	80	90	3	Trace
	French-fried, piece 2 by ½ by ½ inch:						
187	Cooked in deep fat, ready to eat.	10 pieces	57	45	155	2	7
188	Frozen, ready to heat for serving.	10 pieces	57	64	95	2	4
	Mashed:						
189	Milk added	1 cup	195	80	145	4	1
190	Milk and butter added	1 cup	195	76	230	4	12
191	Potato chips, medium, 2-inch-diameter.	10 chips	20	3	110	1	7
192	Pumpkin, canned	1 cup	228	90	75	2	1
193	Radishes, raw, small, without tops.	4 radishes	40	94	10	Trace	Trace
194	Sauerkraut, canned, drained solids.	1 cup	150	91	30	2	Trace
	Spinach:						
195	Cooked	1 cup	180	91	45	6	1
196	Canned, drained solids	1 cup	180	91	45	6	1
197	Canned, strained and creamed.	1 ounce	28	90	10	1	Trace
	Sprouts, raw:						
198	Mung bean	1 cup	90	92	20	3	Trace
199	Soybean	1 cup	107	86	50	7	1
	Squash:						
	Cooked:						
200	Summer, diced	1 cup	210	95	35	1	Trace
201	Winter, baked, mashed	1 cup	205	86	95	4	1
202	Canned, winter, strained or chopped.	1 ounce	28	92	10	Trace	Trace

Fatty acids			Carbohydrate	Calcium	Iron	Vitamin A value	Thiamine	Riboflavin	Niacin	Ascorbic acid
Saturated (total)	Unsaturated									
	Oleic	Linoleic								
Grams	Grams	Grams	Grams	Milligrams	Milligrams	International Units	Milligrams	Milligrams	Milligrams	Milligrams
------	------	------	23	10	0.8	Trace	0.13	0.05	2.0	22
------	------	------	21	9	.7	Trace	.11	.04	1.4	20
2	1	4	20	9	.7	Trace	.06	.04	1.8	8
1	1	2	15	4	.8	Trace	.08	.01	1.2	10
------	------	------	30	47	1.0	50	.17	.11	.2	17
7	4	Trace	28	45	1.0	470	.16	.10	1.6	16
2	2	4	10	6	.4	Trace	.04	.02	.6	2
------	------	------	18	46	1.6	7,750	.04	.14	1.2	------
------	------	------	2	15	.4	10	.01	.01	.1	10
------	------	------	7	54	.8	60	.05	.10	.2	24
------	------	------	6	[4]223	3.6	21,200	.14	.36	1.1	54
------	------	------	6	[4]223	3.6	13,740	.04	.21	.7	26
------	------	------	2	[4]19	.3	750	.01	.03	.1	1
------	------	------	4	26	.7	10	.06	.08	.5	14
------	------	------	6	51	1.1	190	.24	.21	.9	14
------	------	------	8	32	.8	550	.08	.15	1.3	23
------	------	------	23	49	1.6	12,690	.10	.31	1.2	14
------	------	------	2	7	.1	510	.01	.01	.1	1

	Sweetpotatoes:						
	Cooked, medium, 5 by 2 inches, weight raw about 6 ounces:						
203	Baked, peeled after baking.	1 sweetpotato.	110__	64	155	2	1
204	Boiled, peeled after boiling.	1 sweetpotato.	147__	71	170	2	1
205	Candied, 3½ by 2¼ inches__	1 sweetpotato.	175__	60	295	2	6
206	Canned, vacuum or solid pack.	1 cup_____	218__	72	235	4	Trace
	Tomatoes:						
207	Raw, medium, 2 by 2½ inches, about 3 per pound.	1 tomato_____	150__	94	30	2	Trace
208	Canned or cooked_____	1 cup_____	242__	94	45	2	Trace
209	Tomato juice, canned_____	1 cup_____	242__	94	50	2	Trace
210	Tomato catsup_____	1 tablespoon__	17___	70	15	Trace	Trace
211	Turnips, cooked, diced_____	1 cup_____	155__	92	40	1	Trace
	Turnip greens:						
	Cooked:						
212	In small amount of water, short time.	1 cup_____	145__	90	45	4	1
213	In large amount of water, long time.	1 cup_____	145__	90	45	4	1
214	Canned, solids and liquid___	1 cup_____	232__	94	40	3	1

FRUITS AND FRUIT PRODUCTS

215	Apples, raw, medium, 2½-inch-diameter, about 3 per pound.	1 apple_____	150__	85	70	Trace	Trace
216	Apple brown betty_____	1 cup_____	230__	64	350	4	8
217	Applejuice, fresh or canned___	1 cup_____	249__	86	125	Trace	0
	Applesauce, canned:						
218	Sweetened_____	1 cup_____	254__	80	185	Trace	Trace
219	Unsweetened_____	1 cup_____	239__	88	100	Trace	Trace
	Apricots:						
220	Raw, about 12 per pound__	3 apricots____	114__	85	55	1	Trace
	Canned in heavy sirup:						
221	Halves and sirup_____	1 cup_____	259__	77	220	2	Trace
222	Halves, medium, and sirup.	4 halves; 2 tablespoons sirup.	122__	77	105	1	Trace
	Dried:						
223	Uncooked, 40 halves, small.	1 cup_____	150__	25	390	8	1
224	Cooked, unsweetened, fruit and liquid.	1 cup_____	285__	76	240	5	1

4 Calcium may not be usable because of presence of oxalic acid.

-----	-----	-----	36	44	1.0	8,970	.10	.07	.7	24
-----	-----	-----	39	47	1.0	11,610	.13	.09	.9	25
2	3	1	60	65	1.6	11,030	.10	.08	.8	17
-----	-----	-----	54	54	1.7	17,110	.12	.09	1.1	30
-----	-----	-----	6	16	.9	1,640	.08	.06	.8	35
-----	-----	-----	9	27	1.5	2,540	.14	.08	1.7	40
-----	-----	-----	10	17	1.0	2,540	.12	.07	1.8	38
-----	-----	-----	4	2	.1	320	.02	.01	.4	2
-----	-----	-----	9	62	.8	Trace	.06	.09	.6	28
-----	-----	-----	8	376	3.5	15,370	.09	.59	1.0	87
-----	-----	-----	8	376	3.5	15,370	.07	.52	.9	65
-----	-----	-----	7	232	3.7	10,210	.03	.21	1.3	45
-----	-----	-----	18	8	.4	50	.04	.02	.1	3
4	3	Trace	69	41	1.4	270	.13	.10	.9	Trace
-----	-----	-----	34	15	1.2	90	.05	.07	Trace	2
-----	-----	-----	50	10	1.0	80	.05	.03	.1	3
-----	-----	-----	26	10	1.0	70	.05	.02	.1	3
-----	-----	-----	14	18	.5	2,890	.03	.04	.7	10
-----	-----	-----	57	28	.8	4,520	.05	.06	.9	10
-----	-----	-----	27	13	.4	2,130	.02	.03	.4	5
-----	-----	-----	100	100	8.2	16,390	.02	.24	4.9	19
-----	-----	-----	62	63	5.1	10,130	.01	.13	2.8	8

Food, approximate measure, and weight (in grams)			Water	Food energy	Protein	Fat (total lipid)

FRUITS—Continued

			Grams	Per-cent	Calo-ries	Grams	Grams
225	Apricots and applesauce, canned (strained or chopped).	1 ounce	28	80	20	Trace	Trace
226	Apricot nectar	1 cup	250	85	140	1	Trace
	Avocados, raw:						
	California varieties, mainly Fuerte:						
227	10-ounce avocado, about 3⅛ by 4¼ inches, peeled, pitted.	½ avocado	108	74	185	2	18
228	½-inch cubes	1 cup	152	74	260	3	26
	Florida varieties:						
229	13-ounce avocado, about 4 by 3 inches, peeled, pitted.	½ avocado	123	78	160	2	14
230	½-inch cubes	1 cup	152	78	195	2	17
231	Bananas, raw, 6 by 1½ inches, about 3 per pound.	1 banana	150	76	85	1	Trace
232	Blackberries, raw	1 cup	144	85	85	2	1
233	Blueberries, raw	1 cup	140	83	85	1	1
234	Cantaloups, raw, medium, 5-inch-diameter, about 1⅔ pounds.	½ melon	385	94	40	1	Trace
	Cherries:						
235	Raw, sour, sweet, hybrid	1 cup	114	83	65	1	1
236	Canned, red, sour, pitted	1 cup	247	88	105	2	1
237	Cranberry juice cocktail, canned.	1 cup	250	85	140	Trace	Trace
238	Cranberry sauce, sweetened, canned or cooked.	1 cup	277	48	550	Trace	1
239	Dates, "fresh" and dried, pitted, cut.	1 cup	178	20	505	4	1

Fatty acids			Carbo-hy-drate	Cal-cium	Iron	Vita-min A value	Thia-mine	Ribo-flavin	Nia-cin	Ascor-bic acid
Satu-rated (total)	Unsaturated									
	Oleic	Lino-leic								
Grams	Grams	Grams	Grams	Milli-grams	Milli-grams	Inter-national Units	Milli-grams	Milli-grams	Milli-grams	Milli-grams
-----	-----	-----	5·	3	0.2	440	0.01	0.01	0.1	Trace
-----	-----	-----	36	22	.5	2,380	.02	.02	.5	7
4	8	2	6	11	.6	310	.12	.21	1.7	15
5	12	3	9	15	.9	430	.16	.30	2.4	2
3	6	2	11	12	.7	350	.13	.24	2.0	17
3	8	2	13	15	.9	430	.16	.30	2.4	21
-----	-----	-----	23	8	.7	190	.05	.06	.7	10
-----	-----	-----	19	46	1.3	290	.05	.06	.5	30
-----	-----	-----	21	21	1.4	140	.04	.08	.6	20
-----	-----	-----	9	33	.8	[5] 6,590	.09	.07	1.0	63
-----	-----	-----	15	19	.4	650	.05	.06	.4	9
-----	-----	-----	26	37	.7	1,680	.07	.06	.4	13
-----	-----	-----	36	10	.5	20	.02	.02	.1	5
-----	-----	-----	142	22	.8	80	.06	.06	.3	5
-----	-----	-----	134	105	5.7	100	.16	.17	3.9	0

	Figs:						
240	Raw, small, 1½-inch-diameter, about 12 per pound.	3 figs_____	114__	78	90	2	Trace
241	Dried, large, 2 by 1 inch___	1 fig_____	21___	23	60	1	Trace
242	Fruit cocktail, canned in heavy sirup, solids and liquid.	1 cup_____	256__	80	195	1	1
	Grapefruit:						
	Raw, medium, 4¼-inch-diameter, size 64:						
243	White_____	½ grapefruit__	285__	89	50	1	Trace
244	Pink or red_____	½ grapefruit__	285__	89	55	1	Trace
245	Raw sections, white_____	1 cup_____	194__	89	75	1	Trace
	Canned:						
246	Sirup pack, solids and liquid.	1 cup_____	249__	81	170	1	Trace
247	Water pack, solids and liquid.	1 cup_____	240__	91	70	1	Trace
	Grapefruit juice:						
248	Fresh_____	1 cup_____	246__	90	95	1	Trace
	Canned:						
249	Unsweetened_____	1 cup_____	247__	89	100	1	Trace
250	Sweetened_____	1 cup_____	250__	86	130	1	Trace
	Frozen, concentrate, unsweetened:						
251	Undiluted, can, 6 fluid ounces.	1 can_____	207__	62	300	4	1
252	Water added_____	1 cup_____	247__	89	100	1	Trace
	Frozen, concentrate, sweetened:						
253	Undiluted, can, 6 fluid ounces.	1 can_____	211__	57	350	3	1
254	Water added_____	1 cup_____	249__	88	115	1	Trace
	Dehydrated:						
255	Crystals, can, net weight 4 ounces.	1 can_____	114__	1	430	5	1
256	Water added_____	1 cup_____	247__	90	100	1	Trace
	Grapes, raw:						
257	American type (slip skin), such as Concord, Delaware, Niagara, and Scuppernong.	1 cup_____	153__	82	70	1	1
258	European type (adherent skin), such as Malaga, Muscat, Sultanina (Thompson Seedless), and Flame Tokay.	1 cup_____	160__	81	100	1	Trace
259	Grape juice, bottled_____	1 cup_____	254__	83	165	1	Trace

[5] Vitamin A value is based on deeply colored yellow varieties.

-----	-----	-----	22	62	.7	90	.06	.06	.6	2
-----	-----	-----	15	40	.7	20	.02	.02	.1	0
-----	-----	-----	50	23	1.0	360	.04	.03	1.1	5
-----	-----	-----	14	21	.5	10	.05	.02	.2	50
-----	-----	-----	14	21	.5	590	.05	.02	.2	48·
-----	-----	-----	20	31	.8	20	.07	.03	.3	72
-----	-----	-----	44	32	.7	20	.07	.04	.5	75
-----	-----	-----	18	31	.7	20	.07	.04	.5	72
-----	-----	-----	23	22	.5	20	.09	.04	.4	92
-----	-----	-----	24	20	1.0	20	.07	.04	.4	84
-----	-----	-----	32	20	1.0	20	.07	.04	.4	78
-----	-----	-----	72	70	.8	60	.29	.12	1.4	286
-----	-----	-----	24	25	.2	20	.10	.04	.5	96
-----	-----	-----	85	59	.6	50	.24	.11	1.2	245
-----	-----	-----	28	20	.2	20	.08	.03	.4	82
-----	-----	-----	103	99	1.1	90	.41	.18	2.0	399
-----	-----	-----	24	22	.2	20	.10	.05	.5	92
-----	-----	-----	16	13	.4	100	.05	.03	.3	4
-----	-----	-----	26	18	.6	150	.08	.04	.4	7
-----	-----	-----	42	28	.8	--------	.10	.05	;6	Trace

	Food, approximate measure, and weight (in grams)	Water	Food energy	Protein	Fat (total lipid)
	FRUITS—Continued		Per-cent	Calo-ries	Grams	Grams
		Grams				
260	Lemons, raw, medium, 2⅕- 1 lemon_____ 106__ inch-diameter, size 150.	90	20	1	Trace
	Lemon juice:				
261	Fresh_____ 1 cup_____ 246__	91	60	1	Trace
262	1 tablespoon__ 15___	91	5	Trace	Trace
263	Canned, unsweetened_____ 1 cup_____ 245__	92	60	1	Trace
	Lemonade concentrate, frozen, sweetened:				
264	Undiluted, can, 6 fluid 1 can_____ 220__ ounces.	48	430	Trace	Trace
265	Water added_____ 1 cup_____ 248__	88	110	Trace	Trace
	Lime juice:				
266	Fresh_____ 1 cup_____ 246__	90	65	1	Trace
267	Canned_____ 1 cup_____ 246__	90	65	1	Trace
	Limeade concentrate, frozen, sweetened:				
268	Undiluted, can, 6 fluid 1 can_____ 218__ ounces.	50	405	Trace	Trace
269	Water added_____ 1 cup_____ 248__	89	105	Trace	Trace
	Oranges, raw:				
270	Navel, California (winter), 1 orange_____ 180__ size 88, 2⅘-inch-diameter.	85	60	2	Trace
271	Other varieties, 3-inch-diam- 1 orange_____ 210__ eter.	86	70	1	Trace
	Orange juice:				
	Fresh:				
272	California, Valencia, sum- 1 cup_____ 249__ mer.	88	120	2	1
	Florida varieties:				
273	Early and midseason___ 1 cup_____ 247__	90	100	1	Trace
274	Late season, Valencia__ 1 cup_____ 248__	88	110	1	Trace
275	Canned, unsweetened_____ 1 cup_____ 249__	87	120	2	Trace
	Frozen concentrate:				
276	Undiluted, can, 6 fluid 1 can_____ 210__ ounces.	58	330	5	Trace

Fatty acids			Carbo-hy-drate	Cal-cium	Iron	Vita-min A value	Thia-mine	Ribo-flavin	Nia-cin	Ascor-bic acid
Satu-rated (total)	Unsaturated									
	Oleic	Lino-leic								
Grams	Grams	Grams	Grams	Milli-grams	Milli-grams	Inter-national Units	Milli-grams	Milli-grams	Milli-grams	Milli-grams
------	------	------	6	18	0.4	10	0.03	0.01	0.1	38
------	------	------	20	17	.5	40	.08	.03	.2	113
------	------	------	1	1	Trace	Trace	Trace	Trace	Trace	7
------	------	------	19	17	.5	40	.07	.03	.2	102
------	------	------	112	9	.4	40	.05	.06	.7	66
------	------	------	28	2	.1	10	.01	.01	.2	17
------	------	------	22	22	.5	30	.05	.03	.3	80
------	------	------	22	22	.5	30	.05	.03	.3	52
------	------	------	108	11	.7	Trace	.02	.02	.2	262
------	------	------	27	2	.2	Trace	.01	Trace	Trace	6
------	------	------	16	49	.5	240	.12	.05	.5	75
------	------	------	18	63	.3	290	.12	.03	.4	66
------	------	------	26	27	.7	500	.22	.06	.9	122
------	------	------	23	25	.5	490	.22	.06	.9	127
------	------	------	26	25	.5	500	.22	.06	.9	92
------	------	------	28	25	1.0	500	.17	.05	.6	100
------	------	------	80	69	.8	1,490	.63	.10	2.4	332

277	Water added_____	1 cup_____	248__	88	110	2	Trace
278	Dehydrated: Crystals, can, net weight 4 ounces.	1 can_____	113__	1	430	6	2
279	Water added_____	1 cup_____	248__	88	115	1	Trace
280	Orange and grapefruit juice: Frozen concentrate: Undiluted, can, 6 fluid ounces.	1 can_____	209__	59	330	4	1
281	Water added_____	1 cup_____	248__	88	110	1	Trace
282	Papayas, raw, ½-inch cubes__	1 cup_____	182__	89	70	1	Trace
283	Peaches: Raw: Whole, medium, 2-inch- diameter, about 4 per pound.	1 peach_____	114__	89	35	1	Trace
284	Sliced_____	1 cup_____	168__	89	65	1	Trace
285	Canned, yellow-fleshed, solids and liquid: Sirup pack, heavy: Halves or slices_____	1 cup_____	257__	79	200	1	Trace
286	Halves, medium, and sirup.	2 halves and 2 table- spoons sirup.	117__	79	90	Trace	Trace
287	Water pack_____	1 cup_____	245__	91	75	1	Trace
288	Strained_____	1 ounce_____	28___	82	20	Trace	Trace
289	Dried: Uncooked_____	1 cup_____	160__	25	420	5	1
290	Cooked, unsweetened, 10– 12 halves and 6 table- spoons liquid.	1 cup_____	270__	77	220	3	1
291	Frozen: Carton, 12 ounces_____	1 carton_____	340__	79	265	1	Trace
292	Can, 16 ounces_____	1 can_____	454__	79	355	2	Trace
293	Peach nectar, canned_____	1 cup_____	250__	87	115	Trace	Trace
294	Pears: Raw, 3 by 2½-inch-diame- ter.	1 pear_____	182__	83	100	1	1
295	Canned, solids and liquid: Sirup pack, heavy: Halves or slices_____	1 cup_____	255__	80	195	1	1
296	Halves, medium, and sirup.	2 halves and 2 tablespoons sirup.	117__	80	90	Trace	Trace

6 Vitamin A value of yellow-fleshed varieties; the value is negligible in white-fleshed varieties.

------	------	------	27	22	.2	500	.21	.03	.8	112
------	------	------	100	95	1.9	1,900	.76	.24	3.3	406
------	------	------	27	25	.5	500	.20	.06	.9	108
------	------	------	78	61	.8	790	.47	.06	2.3	301
------	------	------	26	20	.2	270	.16	.02	.8	102
------	------	------	18	36	.5	3,190	.07	.08	.5	102
------	------	------	10	9	.5	6 1,320	.02	.05	1.0	7
------	------	------	16	15	.8	6 2,230	.03	.08	1.6	12
------	------	------	52	10	.8	1,100	.02	.06	1.4	7
------	------	------	24	5	.4	500	.01	.03	.7	3
------	------	------	20	10	.7	1,100	.02	.06	1.4	7
------	------	------	5	2	.2	150	Trace	.01	.2	Trace
------	------	------	109	77	9.6	6,240	.02	.31	8.5	28
------	------	------	58	41	5.1	3,300	.01	.15	4.2	6
------	------	------	69	20	1.4	1,770	.04	.10	1.8	7 99
------	------	------	92	27	1.8	2,360	.05	.14	2.4	7 132
------	------	------	31	10	.5	1,070	.02	.05	1.0	1
------	------	------	25	13	.5	30	.04	.07	.2	7
------	------	------	50	13	.5	Trace	.03	.05	.3	4
------	------	------	23	6	.2	Trace	.01	.02	.2	2

7 Content of frozen peaches with added ascorbic acid; when not added the content is 14 milligrams per 12-ounce carton and 18 milligrams per 16-ounce can.

Food, approximate measure, and weight (in grams)			Water	Food energy	Protein	Fat (total lipid)

FRUITS—Continued

			Grams	Per cent	Calories	Grams	Grams
	Pears, canned, solids and liquid—Continued						
297	Water pack_____	1 cup_____	243__	91	80	Trace	Trace
298	Strained_____	1 ounce_____	28___	84	15	Trace	Trace
299	Pear nectar, canned_____	1 cup_____	250__	86	130	1	Trace
300	Persimmons, Japanese or Kaki, raw, seedless, 2½-inch-diameter.	1 persimmon__	125__	79	75	1	Trace
	Pineapple:						
301	Raw, diced_____	1 cup_____	140__	85	75	1	Trace
	Canned, sirup pack, solids and liquid:						
302	Crushed_____	1 cup_____	260__	78	205	1	Trace
303	Sliced, slices and juice___	2 small or 1 large and 2 tablespoons juice.	122__	78	95	Trace	Trace
304	Pineapple juice, canned_____	1 cup_____	249__	86	120	1	Trace
	Plums, all except prunes:						
305	Raw, 2-inch-diameter, about 2 ounces.	1 plum_____	60___	86	30	Trace	Trace
	Canned, sirup pack (Italian prunes):						
306	Plums and juice_____	1 cup_____	256__	79	185	1	Trace
307	Plums (without pits) and juice.	3 plums and 2 tablespoons juice.	122__	79	90	Trace	Trace
	Prunes, dried:						
	Medium, 50–60 per pound:						
308	Uncooked_____	4 prunes_____	32___	24	70	1	Trace
309	Cooked, unsweetened, 17–18 prunes and ⅓ cup liquid.	1 cup_____	270__	65	305	3	1
310	Canned, strained_____	1 ounce_____	28___	73	25	Trace	Trace
311	Prune juice, canned_____	1 cup_____	240__	80	170	1	Trace
312	Raisins, dried_____	1 cup_____	160__	18	460	4	Trace

Fatty acids			Carbohydrate	Calcium	Iron	Vitamin A value	Thiamine	Riboflavin	Niacin	Ascorbic acid
Saturated (total)	Unsaturated									
	Oleic	Linoleic								
Grams	Grams	Grams	Grams	Milligrams	Milligrams	International Units	Milligrams	Milligrams	Milligrams	Milligrams
-----	-----	-----	20	12	0.5	Trace	0.02	0.05	0.3	4
-----	-----	-----	4	3	.1	Trace	Trace	.01	.1	Trace
-----	-----	-----	33	8	.2	10	.01	.05	Trace	1
-----	-----	-----	20	6	.4	2,740	.03	.02	.1	11
-----	-----	-----	19	22	.4	180	.12	.04	.3	33
-----	-----	-----	55	75	1.6	210	.20	.04	.4	23
-----	-----	-----	26	35	.7	100	.09	.02	.2	11
-----	-----	-----	32	37	1.2	200	.13	.04	.4	22
-----	-----	-----	7	10	.3	200	.04	.02	.3	3
-----	-----	-----	50	20	2.7	560	.07	.06	.9	3
-----	-----	-----	25	10	1.3	280	.03	.03	.5	1
-----	-----	-----	19	14	1.0	430	.02	.05	.4	1
-----	-----	-----	81	60	4.5	1,850	.08	.19	1.8	3
-----	-----	-----	7	8	.4	170	.01	.01	.2	1
-----	-----	-----	45	34	9.8	-------	.01	.03	1.1	4
-----	-----	-----	124	99	5.6	30	.18	.13	.9	2

	Raspberries, red:						
313	Raw_____	1 cup_____	123__	84	70	1	1
314	Frozen, 10-ounce carton_____	1 carton_____	284__	74	280	2	1
315	Rhubarb, cooked, sugar added_	1 cup_____	272__	63	385	1	Trace
	Strawberries:						
316	Raw, capped__._____	1 cup_____	149__	90	55	1	1
317	Frozen, 10-ounce carton_____	1 carton_____	284__	72	300	2	1
318	Frozen, 16-ounce can_____	1 can_____	454__	72	485	3	2
319	Tangerines, raw, medium, 2½-inch-diameter, about 4 per pound.	1 tangerine___	114__	87	40	1	Trace
	Tangerine juice:						
320	Canned, unsweetened_____	1 cup_____	248__	89	105	1	Trace
	Frozen concentrate:						
321	Undiluted, can, 6 fluid ounces.	1 can_____	210__	58	340	4	1
322	Water added_____	1 cup_____	248__	88	115	1	Trace
323	Watermelon, raw, wedge, 4 by 8 inches (⅟₁₆ of 10- by 16-inch melon, about 2 pounds with rind).	1 wedge_____	925__	92	120	2	1

GRAIN PRODUCTS

324	Barley, pearled, light, un-cooked.	1 cup_____	203__	11	710	17	2
325	Biscuits, baking powder, with enriched flour, 2½-inch-diameter.	1 biscuit_____	38___	28	130	3	4
326	Bran flakes (40 percent bran) with added thiamine.	1 ounce_____	28___	4	85	3	1
	Breads:						
327	Boston brown bread, made with degermed cornmeal, slice, 3 by ¾ inch.	1 slice_____	48___	45	100	3	1
	Cracked-wheat bread:						
328	Loaf, 1-pound, 20 slices__	1 loaf_____	454__	35	1,190	39	10
329	Slice_____	1 slice_____	23___	35	60	2	1
	French or vienna bread:						
330	Enriched, 1-pound loaf___	1 loaf_____	454__	31	1,315	41	14
331	Unenriched, 1-pound loaf_	1 loaf_____	454__	31	1,315	41	14
	Italian bread:						
332	Enriched, 1-pound loaf___	1 loaf_____	454__	32	1,250	41	4
333	Unenriched, 1-pound loaf_	1 loaf_____	454__	32	1,250	41	4

4 Calcium may not be usable because of presence of oxalic acid.

-----	-----	-----	17	27	1.1	160	.03	.09	.9	31
-----	-----	-----	70	79	1.7	220	.03	.12	.5	45
-----	-----	-----	98	4 112	1.1	70	.02	-----	.2	17
-----	-----	-----	13	31	1.5	90	.04	.10	.9	87
-----	-----	-----	75	62	1.7	120	.05	.14	.5	116
-----	-----	-----	121	100	2.7	190	.08	.23	.8	186
-----	-----	-----	10	34	.3	360	.05	.01	.1	26
-----	-----	-----	25	45	.5	1,050	.14	.04	.3	56
-----	-----	-----	80	130	1.5	3,070	.43	.12	.9	202
-----	-----	-----	27	45	.5	1,020	.14	.04	.3	67
-----	-----	-----	29	30	.9	2,530	.20	.22	.7	26
Trace	1	1	160	32	4.1	0	.25	.17	6.3	0
1	2	Trace	18	61	.7	Trace	.09	.09	.7	Trace
-----	-----	-----	22	17	1.1	0	.13	.07	2.5	0
-----	-----	-----	22	43	.9	0	.05	.03	.6	0
2	5	2	236	399	5.0	Trace	.53	.42	5.8	Trace
-----	-----	-----	12	20	.3	Trace	.03	.02	.3	Trace
3	8	2	251	195	10.0	Trace	1.26	.98	11.3	Trace
3	8	2	251	195	3.2	Trace	.39	.39	3.6	Trace
1	1	2	256	77	10.0	0	1.31	.93	11.7	0
1	1	2	256	77	3.2	0	.39	.27	3.6	0

Food, approximate measure, and weight (in grams)			Water	Food energy	Protein	Fat (total lipid)
GRAIN PRODUCTS—Continued						
Breads—Continued			*Percent*	*Calories*		
Raisin bread:		*Grams*			*Grams*	*Grams*
334	Loaf, 1-pound, 20 slices__	1 loaf_____ 454__	35	1,190	30	13
335	Slice_____	1 slice_____ 23___	35	60	2	1
	Rye bread:					
	American, light (⅓ rye, ⅔ wheat):					
336	Loaf, 1-pound, 20 slices_	1 loaf_____ 454__	36	1,100	41	5
337	Slice_____	1 slice_____ 23___	36	55	2	Trace
338	Pumpernickel, dark, loaf, 1 pound.	1 loaf_____ 454__	34	1,115	41	5
	White bread, enriched: [8]					
	1 to 2 percent nonfat dry milk:					
339	Loaf, 1-pound, 20 slices_	1 loaf_____ 454__	36	1,225	39	15
340	Slice_____	1 slice_____ 23___	36	60	2	1
	3 to 4 percent nonfat dry milk:					
341	Loaf, 1-pound_____	1 loaf_____ 454__	36	1,225	39	15
342	Slice, 20 per loaf____	1 slice_____ 23___	36	60	2	1
343	Slice, toasted_____	1 slice_____ 20___	24	60	2	1
344	Slice, 26 per loaf____	1 slice_____ 17___	36	45	1	1
	5 to 6 percent nonfat dry milk:					
345	Loaf, 1-pound, 20 slices_	1 loaf_____ 454__	35	1,245	41	17
346	Slice_____	1 slice_____ 23___	35	65	2	1
	White bread, unenriched: [8]					
	1 to 2 percent nonfat dry milk:					
347	Loaf, 1-pound, 20 slices_	1 loaf_____ 454__	36	1,225	39	15
348	Slice_____	1 slice_____ 23___	36	60	2	1
	3 to 4 percent nonfat dry milk:					
349	Loaf, 1-pound_____	1 loaf_____ 454__	36	1,225	39	15
350	Slice, 20 per loaf____	1 slice_____ 23___	36	60	2	1
351	Slice, toasted_____	1 slice_____ 20___	24	60	2	1
352	Slice, 26 per loaf____	1 slice_____ 17___	36	45	1	1

Fatty acids			Carbo-hydrate	Cal-cium	Iron	Vita-min A value	Thia-mine	Ribo-flavin	Nia-cin	Ascor-bic acid
Satu-rated (total)	Unsaturated									
	Oleic	Lino-leic								
Grams	Grams	Grams	Grams	Milli-grams	Milli-grams	Inter-national Units	Milli-grams	Milli-grams	Milli-grams	Milli-grams
3	8	2	243	322	5.9	Trace	0.24	0.42	3.0	Trace
------	------	------	12	16	.3	Trace	.01	.02	.2	Trace
1	2	2	236	340	7.3	0	.81	.33	6.4	0
------	------	------	12	17	.4	0	.04	.02	.3	0
1	2	2	241	381	10.9	0	1.05	.63	5.4	0
3	9	2	229	318	10.9	Trace	1.13	.77	10.4	Trace
------	------	------	12	16	.6	Trace	.06	.04	.5	Trace
3	9	2	229	381	11.3	Trace	1.13	.95	10.8	Trace
------	------	------	12	19	.6	Trace	.06	.05	.6	Trace
------	------	------	12	19	.6	Trace	.05	.05	.6	Trace
------	------	------	9	14	.4	Trace	.04	.04	.4	Trace
4	10	2	228	435	11.3	Trace	1.22	.91	11.0	Trace
------	------	------	12	22	.6	Trace	.06	.05	.6	Trace
3	9	2	229	318	3.2	Trace	.40	.36	5.6	Trace
------	------	------	12	16	.2	Trace	.02	.02	.3	Trace
3	9	2	229	381	3.2	Trace	.31	.39	5.0	Trace
------	------	------	12	19	.2	Trace	.02	.02	.3	Trace
------	------	------	12	19	.2	Trace	.01	.02	.3	Trace
------	------	------	9	14	.1	Trace	.01	.01	.2	Trace

	5 to 6 percent nonfat dry milk:						
353	Loaf, 1-pound, 20 slices_	1 loaf_____	454__	35	1,245	41	17
354	Slice_____	1 slice_____	23___	35	65	2	1
	Whole-wheat, graham, entire-wheat bread:						
355	Loaf, 1-pound, 20 slices__	1 loaf_____	454__	36	1,105	48	14
356	Slice_____	1 slice_____	23___	36	55	2	1
357	Toast_____	1 slice_____	19___	24	55	2	1
358	Breadcrumbs, dry, grated____	1 cup_____	88___	6	345	11	4
	Cakes:						
359	Angel food cake; sector, 2-inch (1/12 of 8-inch-diameter cake).	1 sector_____	40___	32	110	3	Trace
360	Chocolate cake, fudge icing; sector, 2-inch (1/16 of 10-inch-diameter layer cake).	1 sector_____	120__	24	420	5	14
361	Fruitcake, dark; piece, 2 by 2 by 1/2 inch.	1 piece_____	30___	23	105	2	4
362	Gingerbread; piece, 2 by 2 by 2 inches.	1 piece_____	55___	30	180	2	7
	Plain cake and cupcakes, without icing:						
363	Piece, 3 by 2 by 1½ inches_	1 piece_____	55___	27	180	4	5
364	Cupcake, 2¾-inch-diameter.	1 cupcake____	40___	27	130	3	3
	Plain cake and cupcakes, with icing:						
365	Sector, 2-inch (1/16 of 10-inch layer cake).	1 sector_____	100__	25	320	5	6
366	Cupcake, 2¾-inch-diameter.	1 cupcake____	50___	25	160	3	3
367	Pound cake; slice, 2¾ by 3 by 5/8 inch.	1 slice_____	30___	19	130	2	7
368	Sponge cake; sector, 2-inch (1/12 of 8-inch-diameter cake).	1 sector_____	40___	32	115	3	2
	Cookies:						
369	Plain and assorted, 3-inch-diameter.	1 cooky_____	25___	5	110	2	3

8 When the amount of nonfat dry milk in commercial white bread is unknown, use values for bread with 3 to 4 percent nonfat dry milk.

9 If the fat used in the recipe is butter or fortified margarine, the vitamin A value for chocolate cake with fudge icing will be 520 I.U. per 2-inch sector,

4	10	2	228	435	3.2	Trace	.32	.59	4.1	Trace
-----	-----	-----	12	22	.2	Trace	.02	.03	.2	Trace
3	7	4	216	449	10.4	Trace	1.17	1.03	12.9	Trace
-----	-----	-----	11	23	.5	Trace	.06	.05	.7	Trace
-----	-----	-----	11	23	.5	Trace	.05	.05	.7	Trace
1	2	1	65	107	3.2	Trace	.19	.26	3.1	Trace
-----	-----	-----	23	2	.1	0	Trace	.05	.1	Trace
5	7	1	70	118	.5	[9] 140	.03	.10	.3	Trace
1	2	Trace	17	29	.8	[9] 50	.04	.04	.3	Trace
2	4	Trace	28	63	1.4	50	.02	.05	.6	Trace
1	3	Trace	31	85	.2	[9] 70	.02	.05	.2	Trace
1	2	Trace	23	62	.2	[9] 50	.01	.03	.1	Trace
2	3	Trace	62	117	.4	[9] 90	.02	.07	.2	Trace
1	1	Trace	31	58	.2	[9] 50	.01	.04	.1	Trace
2	4	1	15	16	.5	[9] 100	.04	.05	.3	Trace
1	1	Trace	22	11	.6	[9] 210	.02	.06	.1	Trace
1	2	Trace	19	6	.2	0	.01	.01	.1	0

item 360; 120 I.U. for fruitcake, item 361; for plain cake without icing, 200 I.U. per piece, item 363; 150 I.U. per cupcake, item 364; for plain cake with icing, 280 I.U. per 2-inch sector, item 365; 140 I.U. per cupcake, item 366; and 300 I.U. for pound cake, item 367.

Food, approximate measure, and weight (in grams)			Water	Food energy	Protein	Fat (total lipid)
GRAIN PRODUCTS—Continued						
Cookies—Continued		Grams	Per-cent	Calo-ries	Grams	Grams
370	Fig bars, small_____	1 fig bar_____ 16___	14	55	1	1
371	Corn-cereal mixture (mainly degermed cornmeal), puffed, with added thiamine, niacin, and iron.	1 ounce_____ 28___	3	115	2	1
	Corn flakes, with added thiamine, niacin, and iron:					
372	Plain_____	1 ounce_____ 28___	4	110	2	Trace
373	Presweetened_____	1 ounce_____ 28___	3	110	1	Trace
	Corn grits, white, degermed, cooked:					
374	Enriched_____	1 cup_____ 242__	87	120	3	Trace
375	Unenriched_____	1 cup_____ 242__	87	120	3	Trace
	Cornmeal, white or yellow, dry:					
376	Whole ground_____	1 cup_____ 118__	12	420	11	5
377	Degermed, enriched_____	1 cup_____ 145__	12	525	11	2
378	Corn muffins, made with enriched, degermed cornmeal; muffin, 2¾-inch-diameter.	1 muffin_____ 48___	30	155	4	5
379	Corn, puffed, presweetened, with added thiamine, riboflavin, niacin, and iron.	1 ounce_____ 28___	3	110	1	Trace
380	Corn and soy shreds, with added thiamine and niacin.	1 ounce_____ 28___	4	100	5	Trace
	Crackers:					
381	Graham_____	4 small or 2 medium. 14___	6	55	1	1
382	Saltines, 2 inches square____	2 crackers____ 8____	5	35	1	1
	Soda, plain:					
383	Cracker, 2½ inches square	2 crackers____ 11___	6	45	1	1
384	Oyster crackers_____	10 crackers___ 10___	6	45	1	1
385	Cracker meal_____	1 tablespoon__ 10___	6	45	1	1
386	Doughnuts, cake type_____	1 doughnut___ 32___	19	135	2	7

| Saturated (total) | Unsaturated | | Carbohydrate | Calcium | Iron | Vitamin A value | Thiamine | Riboflavin | Niacin | Ascorbic acid |
	Oleic	Linoleic								
Grams	Grams	Grams	Grams	Milligrams	Milligrams	International Units	Milligrams	Milligrams	Milligrams	Milligrams
-----	-----	-----	12	11	0.2	0	Trace	0.01	0.1	0.
-----	-----	-----	23	6	1.2	--------	.15	.04	.6	0
-----	-----	-----	24	3	.5	--------	.12	.03	.6	0
-----	-----	-----	26	3	.4	--------	.12	.01	.5	0
-----	-----	-----	27	2	.7	Trace	.11	.08	1.0	0
-----	-----	-----	27	2	.2	Trace	.04	.01	.4	0
1	2	2	87	12	2.8	[10] 600	.45	.13	2.4	0
Trace	1	1	114	9	[11] 4.2	[10] 430	[11] .64	[11] .38	[11] 5.1	0
2	2	Trace	22	79	.9	[12] 170	.10	.15	.8	Trace
-----	-----	-----	26	3	.5	--------	.12	.05	.6	0
-----	-----	-----	21	24	1.2	--------	.19	.04	.6	0
-----	-----	-----	10	3	.3	0	.04	.02	.2	0
-----	-----	-----	6	2	.1	0	Trace	Trace	.1	0
-----	-----	-----	8	2	.1	0	.01	.01	.1	0
-----	-----	-----	7	2	.1	0	.01	Trace	.1	0
-----	-----	-----	7	2	.1	0	.01	Trace	.1	0
2	2	3	17	23	.4	40	.05	.04	.4	0

387	Farina, cooked; enriched to minimum levels for required nutrients and for the optional nutrient, calcium.	1 cup_____	238__	89	105	3	Trace
	Macaroni, cooked:						
	Enriched:						
388	Cooked 8–10 minutes (undergoes additional cooking in a food mixture).	1 cup_____	130__	64	190	6	1
389	Cooked until tender_____	1 cup_____	140__	72	155	5	1
	Unenriched:						
390	Cooked 8–10 minutes (undergoes additional cooking in a food mixture).	1 cup_____	130__	64	190	6	1
391	Cooked until tender_____	1 cup_____	140__	72	155	5	1
392	Macaroni, enriched, and cheese, baked.	1 cup_____	220__	58	475	18	25
393	Muffins, with enriched white flour; muffin, 2¾-inch-diameter.	1 muffin_____	48___	39	135	4	5
	Noodles (egg noodles), cooked:						
394	Enriched_____	1 cup_____	160__	70	200	7	2
395	Unenriched_____	1 cup_____	160__	70	200	7	2
396	Oat-cereal mixture, mainly oats, with added B-vitamins and minerals.	1 ounce_____	28___	3	115	4	2
397	Oatmeal or rolled oats, regular or quick-cooking, cooked.	1 cup_____	236__	85	150	5	3
	Pancakes (griddlecakes),4-inch-diameter:						
398	Wheat, enriched flour (home recipe).	1 cake_____	27___	53	60	2	2
399	Buckwheat (buckwheat pancake mix).	1 cake_____	27___	62	45	2	2
	Piecrust, plain, baked:						
	Enriched flour:						
400	Lower crust, 9-inch shell_	1 crust_____	135__	10	655	10	36
401	Double crust, 9-inch pie__	1 double crust_	270__	10	1,315	20	73
	Unenriched flour:						
402	Lower crust, 9-inch shell_	1 crust_____	135__	10	655	10	36
403	Double crust, 9-inch pie__	1 double crust_	270__	10	1,315	20	73

[10] Vitamin A value based on yellow cornmeal; white cornmeal contains only a trace.

[11] Iron, thiamine, riboflavin, and niacin are based on the minimal level of enrichment specified in the standards of identity promulgated under the Federal Food, Drug, and Cosmetic Act.

------	------	------	22	31	.8	0	.11	.07	1.0	0
------	------	------	39	14	1.4	0	.23	.14	1.9	0
------	------	------	32	11	1.3	0	.19	.11	1.5	0
------	------	------	39	14	.6	0	.02	.02	.5	0
------	------	------	32	11	.6	0	.02	.02	.4	0
14	8	1	44	394	2.0	970	.22	.46	1.9	Trace
1	3	Trace	19	74	.7	60	.08	.11	.7	Trace
1	1	Trace	37	16	1.4	60	.23	.14	1.8	0
1	1	Trace	37	16	1.0	60	.04	.03	.7	0
Trace	1	1	21	45	1.2	0	.22	.04	.5	0
1	1	1	26	21	1.7	0	.22	.05	.4	0
Trace	1	Trace	8	34	.3	30	.05	.06	.3	Trace
1	1	Trace	6	67	.3	30	.04	.04	.2	Trace
8	24	3	72	15	2.7	0	.29	.23	3.0	0
17	47	5	143	30	5.4	0	.58	.47	5.9	0
8	24	3	72	15	.7	0	.05	.03	.7	0
17	47	5	143	30	1.4	0	.09	.06	1.4	0

12 Based on recipe using white cornmeal; if yellow cornmeal is used the vitamin A value is 240 I.U.

Food, approximate measure, and weight (in grams)			Water	Food energy	Protein	Fat (total lipid)

GRAIN PRODUCTS—Continued

			Per-cent	Calo-ries	Grams	Grams
	Pies; sector, 4-inch, ⅐ of 9-inch-diameter pie:	*Grams*				
404	Apple	1 sector	135	48	330	3	13
405	Cherry	1 sector	135	46	340	3	13
406	Custard	1 sector	130	58	265	7	11
407	Lemon meringue	1 sector	120	47	300	4	12
408	Mince	1 sector	135	43	340	3	9
409	Pumpkin	1 sector	130	59	265	5	12
410	Pizza (cheese), 5½-inch sector, ⅛ of 14-inch-diameter pie.	1 sector	75	47	180	8	6
411	Popcorn, popped	1 cup	14	4	55	2	1
412	Pretzels, small stick	5 sticks	5	8	20	Trace	Trace
	Rice, cooked:					
413	Parboiled	1 cup	176	72	205	4	Trace
414	White	1 cup	168	71	200	4	Trace
415	Rice, puffed, with added thiamine, niacin, and iron.	1 cup	14	5	55	1	Trace
416	Rice flakes, with added thiamine and niacin.	1 cup	30	5	115	2	Trace
	Rolls:					
	Plain, pan; 12 per 16 ounces:					
417	Enriched	1 roll	38	31	115	3	2
418	Unenriched	1 roll	38	31	115	3	2
419	Hard, round; 12 per 22 ounces.	1 roll	52	25	160	5	2
420	Sweet, pan; 12 per 18 ounces.	1 roll	43	31	135	4	4
421	Rye wafers, 1⅞ by 3½ inches.	2 wafers	13	6	45	2	Trace
	Spaghetti, cooked until tender:					
422	Enriched	1 cup	140	72	155	5	1
423	Unenriched	1 cup	140	72	155	5	1

Fatty acids			Carbo-hy-drate	Cal-cium	Iron	Vita-min A value	Thia-mine	Ribo-flavin	Nia-cin	Ascor-bic acid
Satu-rated (total)	Unsaturated									
	Oleic	Lino-leic								
Grams	Grams	Grams	Grams	Milli-grams	Milli-grams	Inter-national Units	Milli-grams	Milli-grams	Milli-grams	Milli-grams
4	7	1	53	9	0.5	220	0.04	0.02	0.3	1
4	7	1	55	14	.5	520	.04	.02	.3	2
4	6	1	34	162	1.6	290	.07	.21	.4	0
4	6	1	45	24	.6	210	.04	.10	.2	1
2	6	1	62	22	3.0	10	.09	.05	.5	1
5	6	1	34	70	1.0	2,480	.04	.15	.4	0
3	3	Trace	23	157	.7	570	.03	.09	.8	8
------	------	------	11	2	.4	0	.05	.02	.3	0
------	------	------	4	1	0	0	Trace	Trace	Trace	0
------	------	------	45	14	.5	0	.10	.02	1.9	0
------	------	------	44	13	.5	0	.02	.01	.7	0
------	------	------	12	2	.3	--------	.06	.01	.6	0
------	------	------	26	9	.5	--------	.11	.01	1.7	0
1	1	Trace	20	28	.7	Trace	.11	.07	.8	Trace
1	1	Trace	20	28	.3	Trace	.02	.03	.3	Trace
1	1	Trace	31	24	.4	Trace	.03	.05	.4	Trace
1	2	Trace	21	37	.3	30	.03	.06	.4	0
------	------	------	10	6	.6	0	.04	.03	.2	0
------	------	------	32	11	1.3	0	.19	.11	1.5	0
------	------	------	32	11	.6	0	.02	.02	.4	0

424	Spaghetti with meat sauce____	1 cup_____	250__	76	285	13	10
425	Spaghetti in tomato sauce with cheese.	1 cup_____	250__	80	210	6	5
426	Waffles, with enriched flour, ½ by 4½ by 5½ inches.	1 waffle_____	75___	34	240	8	9
	Wheat, puffed:						
427	With added thiamine, niacin, and iron.	1 ounce_____	28___	4	100	4	Trace
428	With added thiamine and niacin; presweetened.	1 ounce_____	28___	3	105	1	Trace
429	Wheat, rolled; cooked_____	1 cup_____	236__	80	175	5	1
430	Wheat, shredded, plain (long, round, or bite-size).	1 ounce_____	28___	6	100	3	1
431	Wheat and malted barley cereal, with added thiamine, niacin, and iron.	1 ounce_____	28___	3	105	3	Trace
432	Wheat flakes, with added thiamine, niacin, and iron.	1 ounce_____	28___	4	100	3	Trace
	Wheat flours:						
433	Whole-wheat, from hard wheats, stirred.	1 cup_____	120__	12	400	16	2
	All-purpose or family flour:						
434	Enriched, sifted_____	1 cup_____	110__	12	400	12	1
435	Unenriched, sifted_____	1 cup_____	110__	12	400	12	1
	Self-rising:						
436	Enriched_____	1 cup_____	110__	12	385	10	1
437	Unenriched_____	1 cup_____	110__	12	385	10	1
438	Wheat germ, stirred_____	1 cup_____	68___	11	245	17	7

FATS, OILS

	Butter, 4 sticks per pound:						
439	Sticks, 2_____	1 cup_____	224__	16	1,605	1	181
440	Stick, ⅛_____	1 tablespoon__	14___	16	100	Trace	11
441	Pat or square (64 per pound)_	1 pat_____	7____	16	50	Trace	6
	Fats, cooking:						
442	Lard_____	1 cup_____	220__	0	1,985	0	220
443		1 tablespoon__	14___	0	135	0	14
444	Vegetable fats_____	1 cup_____	200__	0	1,770	0	200
445		1 tablespoon__	12.5_	0	110	0	12

[11] Iron, thiamine, riboflavin, and niacin are based on the minimal level of enrichment specified in standards of identity promulgated under the Federal Food, Drug, and Cosmetic Act.

3	3	3	35	25	2.0	690	.07	.10	2.1	13
2	1	2	36	45	1.0	830	.07	.08	1.0	15
3	5	1	30	124	1.4	310	.14	.21	1.1	Trace
-----	-----	-----	22	8	1.2	0	.16	.06	2.2	0
-----	-----	-----	26	4	.5	0	.12	.01	1.4	0
-----	-----	-----	40	19	1.7	0	.17	.06	2.1	0
-----	-----	-----	23	13	1.0	0	.06	.03	1.3	0
-----	-----	-----	24	13	1.0	0	.13	.05	1.5	0
-----	-----	-----	23	13	1.2	0	.16	.05	1.8	0
Trace	1	1	85	49	4.0	0	.66	.14	5.2	0
-----	-----	-----	84	18	[11] 3.2	0	[11].48	[11].29	[11] 3.8	0
-----	-----	-----	84	18	.9	0	.07	.05	1.0	0
-----	-----	-----	81	299	[11] 3.2	0	[11].48	[11].29	[11] 3.8	0
			81	299	1.1	0	.08	.05	1.3	0
1	2	3	34	57	5.5	0	1.39	.54	3.1	0
100	60	5	1	45	Trace	[13] 7,400	-----	-----	-----	0
6	4	Trace	Trace	3	Trace	[13] 460	-----	-----	-----	0
3	2	0	Trace	1	Trace	[13] 230	-----	-----	-----	0
84	101	22	0	0	0	0	0	0	0	0
5	6	1	0	0	0	0	0	0	0	0
46	130	14	0	0	0	0	0	0	0	0
3	8	1	0	0	0	0	0	0	0	0

[13] Year-round average.

	Food, approximate measure, and weight (in grams)			Water	Food energy	Protein	Fat (total lipid)
	FATS, OILS—Continued						
	Margarine, 4 sticks per pound:		*Grams*	*Percent*	*Calories*	*Grams*	*Grams*
446	Sticks, 2	1 cup	224	16	1,615	1	181
447	Stick, ⅛	1 tablespoon	14	16	100	Trace	11
448	Pat or square (64 per pound).	1 pat	7	16	50	Trace	6
	Oils, salad or cooking:						
449	Corn	1 tablespoon	14	0	125	0	14
450	Cottonseed	1 tablespoon	14	0	125	0	14
451	Olive	1 tablespoon	14	0	125	0	14
452	Soybean	1 tablespoon	14	0	125	0	14
	Salad dressings:						
453	Blue cheese	1 tablespoon	16	28	90	1	10
454	Commercial, plain; mayonnaise type.	1 tablespoon	15	48	60	Trace	6
455	French	1 tablespoon	15	42	60	Trace	6
456	Home cooked, boiled	1 tablespoon	17	68	30	1	2
457	Mayonnaise	1 tablespoon	15	14	110	Trace	12
458	Thousand Island	1 tablespoon	15	38	75	Trace	8
	SUGARS, SWEETS						
	Candy:						
459	Caramels	1 ounce	28	7	120	1	3
460	Chocolate, sweetened, milk	1 ounce	28	1	145	2	9
461	Fudge, plain	1 ounce	28	5	115	Trace	3
462	Hard candy	1 ounce	28	1	110	0	0
463	Marshmallow	1 ounce	28	15	90	1	0
464	Chocolate sirup	1 tablespoon	20	39	40	Trace	Trace
465	Honey, strained or extracted	1 tablespoon	21	20	60	Trace	0
466	Jams, marmalades, preserves	1 tablespoon	20	28	55	Trace	Trace
467	Jellies	1 tablespoon	20	34	50	0	0

Fatty acids			Carbohydrate	Calcium	Iron	Vitamin A value	Thiamine	Riboflavin	Niacin	Ascorbic acid
Saturated (total)	Unsaturated									
	Oleic	Linoleic								
Grams	Grams	Grams	Grams	Milligrams	Milligrams	International Units	Milligrams	Milligrams	Milligrams	Milligrams
47	103	16	1	45	Trace	[14] 7,400	------	------	------	0
3	6	1	Trace	3	Trace	[14] 460	------	------	------	0
1	3	1	Trace	1	Trace	[14] 230	------	------	------	0
1	4	7	0	0	0	--------	0	0	0	0
3	3	7	0	0	0	--------	0	0	0	0
2	11	1	0	0	0	--------	0	0	0	0
2	3	7	0	0	0	--------	0	0	0	0
2	2	5	1	11	Trace	30	Trace	.02	Trace	Trace
1	1	3	2	2	Trace	30	Trace	Trace	Trace	0
1	1	3	2	3	.1	0	0	0	0	0
1	1	Trace	3	15	.1	80	.01	.03	Trace	Trace
2	3	6	Trace	2	.1	40	Trace	Trace	Trace	0
1	2	4	1	2	.1	60	Trace	Trace	Trace	2
2	1	Trace	22	36	.7	50	.01	.04	Trace	Trace
5	3	Trace	16	61	.3	40	.03	.11	.2	0
2	1	Trace	23	14	.1	60	Trace	.02	Trace	Trace
------	------	------	28	0	0	0	0	0	0	0
------	------	------	23	0	0	0	0	0	0	0
------	------	------	11	3	.3	--------	------	------	------	------
------	------	------	17	1	.2	0	Trace	.01	Trace	1
------	------	------	14	2	.1	Trace	Trace	Trace	Trace	1
------	------	------	13	2	.1	Trace	Trace	Trace	Trace	1

No.	Food	Measure					
	Molasses, cane:						
468	Light (first extraction)_____	1 tablespoon__	20___	24	50	------	------
469	Blackstrap (third extraction)	1 tablespoon__	20___	24	45	------	------
470	Sirup, table blends_____	1 tablespoon__	20___	25	55	0	0
	Sugar:						
471	Granulated, cane or beet___	1 cup_____	200__	Trace	770	0	0
472		1 tablespoon__	12___	Trace	50	0	0
473	Lump, 1⅛ by ⅝ by ⅜ inch__	1 lump_____	7____	Trace	25	0	0
474	Powdered, stirred before measuring.	1 cup_____	128__	Trace	495	0	0
475		1 tablespoon__	8____	Trace	30	0	0
476	Brown, firm-packed_____	1 cup_____	220__	3	815	0	0
477		1 tablespoon__	14___	3	50	0	0

MISCELLANEOUS ITEMS

No.	Food	Measure					
478	Beer (average 4 percent alcohol).	1 cup_____	240__	90	([16])	1	Trace
	Beverages, carbonated:						
479	Ginger ale_____	1 cup_____	230__	91	80	------	------
480	Kola type_____	1 cup_____	230__	88	105	------	------
481	Bouillon cube, ⅝ inch_____	1 cube_____	4____	5	2	Trace	Trace
	Chili powder. See Vegetables, Peppers.						
482	Chili sauce (mainly tomatoes)_	1 tablespoon__	17___	69	15	Trace	Trace
	Chocolate:						
483	Bitter or unsweetened_____	1 ounce_____	28___	2	145	2	15
484	Sweetened_____	1 ounce_____	28___	1	135	1	8
	Cider. See Fruit, Applejuice.						
	Gelatin, dry:						
485	Plain_____	1 tablespoon__	10___	13	35	9	Trace
486	Dessert powder, 3-ounce package.	½ cup_____	85___	2	325	8	Trace
	Gelatin dessert, ready-to-eat:						
487	Plain_____	1 cup_____	239__	83	155	4	Trace
488	With fruit_____	1 cup_____	241__	81	170	3	Trace
	Olives, pickled:						
489	Green_____	12 Extra Large or 7 Jumbo.	66___	78	65	1	7
490	Ripe: Mission; other varieties, such as Ascolano, Manzanillo, and Sevillano.	12 Extra Large or 7 Jumbo.	66___	76	85	1	9

[14] Based on the average vitamin A content of fortified margarine. Federal specifications for fortified margarine require a minimum of 15,000 I.U. of vitamin A per pound.

-----	-----	-----	13	33	.9	--------	.01	.01	Trace	------
-----	-----	-----	11	116	2.3	--------	.02	.04	.3	------
-----	-----	-----	15	9	.8	0	0	Trace	Trace	0
-----	-----	-----	199	------	------	0	0	0	0	0
-----	-----	-----	12	------	------	0	0	0	0	0
-----	-----	-----	7	------	------	0	0	0	0	0
-----	-----	-----	127	------	------	0	0	0	0	0
-----	-----	-----	8	------	------	0	0	0	0	0
-----	-----	-----	210	15 167	5.7	0	0	0	0	0
-----	-----	-----	13	15 10	.4	0	0	0	0	0
-----	-----	-----	11	10	Trace	0	Trace	.06	.4	0
-----	-----	-----	21	------	------	--------	------	------	------	------
-----	-----	-----	28	------	------	--------	------	------	------	------
-----	-----	-----	0	------	------	--------	------	.07	1.0	0
-----	-----	-----	4	2	.1	320	.02	.01	.4	2
8	6	Trace	8	28	1.2	20	.01	.06	.3	0
5	3	Trace	18	18	.8	10	.01	.04	.2	0
-----	-----	-----	0	0	0	0	0	0	0	0
-----	-----	-----	76	0	0	0	0	0	0	0
-----	-----	-----	36	0	0	0	0	0	0	0
-----	-----	-----	42	14	.7	270	.07	.05	.5	7
1	5	Trace	1	48	.9	170	Trace	------	------	------
1	7	1	2	45	.9	40	Trace	Trace	------	------

15 Calcium value is based on dark brown sugar; value is lower for light brown sugar.

16 The value excluding energy derived from alcohol is 48 calories. If the energy from alcohol is considered available, the value is 114 calories.

	Food, approximate measure, and weight (in grams)			Water	Food energy	Protein	Fat (total lipid)
	MISCELLANEOUS ITEMS—Continued						
	Pickles, cucumber:		*Grams*	*Per-cent*	*Calories*	*Grams*	*Grams*
491	Dill, large, 4 by 1¾ inches__	1 pickle_____	135__	93	15	1	Trace
492	Sweet, 2¾ by ¾ inch_____	1 pickle_____	20___	70	20	Trace	Trace
	Popcorn. *See* Grain Products.						
493	Sherbet, factory packed_____	1 cup_____	193__	68	235	3	Trace
	Soups, canned; ready-to-serve:						
494	Bean_____	1 cup_____	250__	82	190	8	5
495	Beef_____	1 cup_____	250__	92	100	6	4
496	Bouillon, broth, consomme_	1 cup_____	240__	95	10	2	_____
497	Chicken_____	1 cup_____	250__	94	75	4	2
498	Clam chowder_____	1 cup_____	255__	91	85	5	2
499	Cream soup (asparagus, celery, mushroom).	1 cup_____	255__	85	200	7	12
500	Noodle, rice, barley_____	1 cup_____	250__	90	115	6	4
501	Pea_____	1 cup_____	245__	86	140	6	2
502	Tomato_____	1 cup_____	245__	91	90	2	2
503	Vegetable_____	1 cup_____	250__	92	80	4	2
504	Starch, pure, including arrowroot, corn, etc.	1 cup_____	128__	12	465	1	Trace
505		1 tablespoon__	8____	12	30	Trace	Trace
506	Tapioca, quick-cooking granulated, dry; stirred before measuring.	1 cup_____	152__	13	545	1	Trace
507		1 tablespoon__	10___	13	35	Trace	Trace
508	Vinegar_____	1 tablespoon__	15___	_____	2	0	_____
509	White sauce, medium_____	1 cup_____	265__	73	430	10	33
	Yeast:						
	Baker's:						
510	Compressed_____	1 ounce_____	28___	71	25	3	Trace
511	Dry active_____	1 ounce_____	28___	5	80	10	Trace
512	Brewer's, dry_____	1 tablespoon__	8____	5	25	3	Trace
	Yoghurt. *See* Milk, Cream, Cheese; Related Products.						

Fatty acids			Carbo-hy-drate	Cal-cium	Iron	Vita-min A value	Thia-mine	Ribo-flavin	Nia-cin	Ascor-bic acid
Satu-rated (total)	Unsaturated									
	Oleic	Lino-leic								
Grams	*Grams*	*Grams*	*Grams*	*Milli-grams*	*Milli-grams*	*Inter-national Units*	*Milli-grams*	*Milli-grams*	*Milli-grams*	*Milli-grams*
------	------	------	3	34	1.6	420	Trace	0.09	0.1	8
------	------	------	5	3	.3	20	0	Trace	Trace	1
------	------	------	58	96	.1	0	.03	.15	.1	0
2	2	Trace	30	95	2.8	--------	.10	.10	.8	------
2	2	Trace	11	15	.5	--------	-----	-----	-----	------
-----	-----	-----	0	2	1.0	0	0	.05	.6	0
1	1	Trace	10	20	.5	--------	.02	.12	1.5	------
Trace	Trace	1	12	36	3.6	--------	-----	-----	-----	------
7	4	Trace	18	217	.5	200	.05	.20	.1	0
1	2	1	13	82	.2	30	.02	.05	.7	0
1	1	Trace	25	32	1.5	440	.17	.07	1.2	5
1	Trace	1	18	24	1.0	1,230	.02	.10	.7	10
1	1	Trace	14	32	.8	--------	.05	.08	1.0	8
------	------	------	111	0	0	0	0	0	0	0
------	------	------	7	0	0	0	0	0	0	0
------	------	------	131	18	1.5	0	0	0	0	0
------	------	------	8	1	.1	0	0	0	0	0
------	------	------	1	1	.1	--------	-----	-----	-----	------
18	11	1	23	305	.3	1,350	.07	.42	.3	1
------	------	------	3	4	1.4	Trace	.20	.47	3.2	Trace
------	------	------	11	12	4.6	Trace	.66	1.53	10.4	Trace
------	------	------	3	17	1.4	Trace	1.25	.34	3.0	Trace

TABLE 2

TABLE 2.—YIELD OF COOKED MEAT PER POUND OF RAW MEAT

Meat as purchased	Yield of cooked meat (without drippings)	
	Description	Approximate weight per pound of raw meat
		Ounces
Chops or steaks for broiling or frying:		
With bone and relatively large amount of fat, such as: Pork or lamb chops; beef rib, sirloin, or porterhouse steaks.	With bone and fat	10–12
	Without bone, with fat	7–10
	Lean only	5–7
Without bone and with very little fat, such as: Round of beef; veal steaks	Lean and fat	12–13
	Lean only	9–12
Ground meat for broiling or frying, market type, such as: Hamburger; lamb or pork patties	Patties	9–13
Roasts for oven cooking (no liquid added):		
With bone and relatively large amount of fat, such as: Beef rib, loin, chuck; lamb shoulder, leg; pork, fresh or cured.	With bone and fat	10–12
	Without bone, with fat	8–10
	Lean only	6–9
Without bone	Lean and fat	10–12
	Lean only	7–10
Cuts for pot-roasting, simmering, braising, stewing:		
With bone and relatively large amount of fat, such as: Beef chuck; pork shoulder	With bone and fat	10–11
	Without bone, with fat	8–9
	Lean only	6–8
Without bone and with relatively small amount of fat, such as: Trimmed beef; veal	Lean with small amount of adhering fat	9–11

APPENDIX H

RETAIL SOURCES OF HEALTH FOODS IN THE UNITED STATES

This list attempts to cover the entire country, but, for reasons beyond the publisher's control, may be incomplete.

ALABAMA

BIRMINGHAM, V. H. Huey
MONTGOMERY, Aldridge Natural Food

ARIZONA

FLAGSTAFF, Flagstaff Natural Health
    Food Town Super Market
GLENDALE, Alvah Health Products
MESA, Lodo's Health Food
PHOENIX, Eichenauer Health Foods
    Grace's Health Kitchen
    Minall Health Products
    Organic Sea Produce of Arizona
    Paradise Health Food Store
    Robert's Health Food Center
    Vitality Health Foods
PINETOP, Dew Drop Inn Mercantile
PRESCOTT, Mac's Food Market
SEDONA, Sun Valley Health Products
    Bopp Health Food Store
TUCSON, Raymond C. Farney
    House of Nutrition
    Nutrition Center of Tucson
YUMA, Messner
    Yuma Health Food Store

ARKANSAS

FAYETTEVILLE, Heart of the Ozarks Health Products
FT. SMITH, Health Food Co.
LITTLE ROCK, Health Food Center
SPRINGDALE, Graham Natural Foods

CALIFORNIA

ALHAMBRA, El Molino Mills
    Mathew's Nutrition Center
    Vita Health Food Center
ANAHEIM, Pacific Health Food Store
    Russell's Health Foods
ARCADIA, Arcadia Coop.
    Arcadia Nutrition Center
ARLINGTON, La Sierra College Store
AUBURN, Hungry Hill Health Foods
BAKERSFIELD, Gay Health Foods
BANNING, K's Food Shop
BEAUMONT, Dona Gray Pure Products
BELL, Bell Dietary Foods
BELLFLOWER, Steven's Health Food Store
BERKELEY, Berkeley Health Foods
    Consumer's Coop.
    Goodson's Health Foods
BEVERLY HILLS, Jones' Health Foods
BURBANK, H. F. Burbank Store
BURLINGAME, Vitality House
CARMEL, Osborne's Nutrition Center
    Sargent's
CARMICHAEL, Elliott's
    Vi's Vital Foods
CASTRO VALLEY, Shirley's Health Food Shop
CHICAGO, Victory Vegetable Formulas
CHICO, Chico Health Food Store
CHULA VISTA, Chula Vista Health Store
    House of Nutrition
COMPTON, Ridenour's
CONTANA, Vitamin Charlie
COOS BAY, George's Food Market
COSTA MESA, Shaw's Nutrition Square

COVINA, Barklow's
CRESCENT CITY, Crescent City Health Foods
CULVER CITY, Culver City Health Food
DESERT HOT SPRINGS, El Pueblo Market
    Snyder's
EL CAJON, Valley Health
EL CENTRO, Tasti Foods
EL MONTE, Crawford's
    El Monte Center
    Hansen's
    Valley Health Food Center
    Vit A Day Nut Store
ELSINORE, Rosenberg's
    Tontz Honey Farm Store
ENCINATOS, Health Food Store
    Your House of Health
ESCONDIDO, Escondido Health
    The Hunza House
EUREKA, Paulsen's House of Better Living
FALLBROOK, Clemon's
FONTANA, Dennell's Health Foods
FRESNO, Dane's Health Foods
    Health Foods Center
    Tower Diet Foods
FULLERTON, California Health Food Store
GARDEN GROVE, Carroll's
GLENDALE, Foods For Life
    Glendale Mercantile Co.
    Nutrition Food Shop
    Oliphant's
    Pacific Union Conference
    Sunset Natural Food Store
GRASS VALLEY, Modern Health Foods
HANFORD, Melvin
HAYWARD, Dorothea's
    Kraski's Nutrition Center
HEMET, Roberts Health Foods
HERMOSA BEACH, South Bay Health Food Store
    Village Health Corner
HOLLYWOOD, Apollo Natural Foods

HUNTINGTON PARK, House of Vitamins
    Seiler's Health Food Mart
INGLEWOOD, Ludwick's Natural Foods
    Sun Vitamins
LA CRESCENTA, La Crescenta Nutrition Service
LAGUNA BEACH, Laguna Health Food Store
    Washbrook's Health Foods
    Welsh's Natural Foods
LA HABRE, Dr. Kear
LA JOLLA, Diet Foods
    La Jolla Health Food
LA MESA, La Mesa Health Food
LAWNDALE, Lawndale Health Food Store
LEMON GROVE, Lemon Grove Healthful Foods
LODI, Buoyant Health Service
LOMA LINDA, Loma Linda Market
LOMITA, Lomita Health Food Store
LONG BEACH, Al Live Longer
    Given's
    Haseltine's Health Foods
    Health Food Center
    Long Beach Health Food Shop
    Long Beach Vegetable Juice Co.
    Moore's Stone Mill
    Naturade Products Inc.
    Old Mill Health Foods
    Schulman's
    Schulman's Nutrition Center
    Sunshine Health Foods
    Vitamin Home
    Ruth G. Walker
LONGMONT, The Corner Pantry
LOS ANGELES, Alfred's
    Apollo Health Foods
    Basic & Dietetic Foods
    Better Food Management
    C. A. Brandman
    Bullock's
    Christ Mill Health Foods
    Colonial Natural Health Foods Store
    Dan's Health Food

Diet House
Farmers Market
Foods Unlimited #5
Foundation Foods
Goebel Health Foods
Good Health Shop
Goodman's
The Grist Mill
Haseltine's
Health Pantry
Hollywood Natural Foods
Hollywood Vitamin House
Mitchel N. Hotra
House of Better Living
House of Vitamins
Jay's Dietary Foods
Jones Grain Mill
Lindberg Nutrition Service
May Company
Miracle Mill Health Foods
Modern House of Health
Oasis of Health
Patton's Products
Pep's Natural Food Store
Redpath Gymnasium
Sanford's
Scientific Foods
Sure Health Foods
Sure Health Store
Vita Food Store
Wilshire Health Center
West Health Food Store
LOS GATOS, Welget Health Center
MERCED, Kay's Health Foods
MILL VALLEY, Mill Valey Health Foods
MODESTO, Dane's
    Healthway Food Center
MONROVIA, Monrovia Health Food
MONTEREY, Healthway House
    Monterey Health Food Center
MONTROSE, Nature's Health Foods

MOUNTAINVIEW, Natural Way Health Center
MT. SHASTA, House of Health
NAPA, Gardner's Health Foods
NATIONAL CITY, George's
    Paradise Valley San.
NEWPORT BEACH, Harbor Health Food
    Richard's Lido Market
NORTH HOLLYWOOD, The Good Life
    Sunset Natural Foods
OAKLAND, F. A. Bray
    California Health Food
    College Avenue Health Foods
    The Food Mill
    Fountain of Health
    Fruitvale Diet Shoppe
    Healthcraft, Inc.
    Hartung's
    Lakeshore Health Foods
    National Consumers Service
    Oakland Health Food Store
    Piedmont Ave. Natural Foods
    Sherman's Health Foods
OCEAN BEACH, 1890 Store
OCEANSIDE, Your Health Food Store
OJAI, R. H. Weldon
ONTARIO, Vita Foods
    Vitanutrition Service
ORANGE, Pacific Shop
PACIFIC GROVE, Grove Nutrition Center
PACIFIC PALISADES, Foods Unlimited #22
    R. M. Friedman
PALM SPRINGS, Palm Springs House of Health
PALO ALTO, Eat-Right Health Foods
    Liddicoat, Inc.
    Palo Alto Health Food
PASADENA, Bee Balser's House of Health
    Health Food House
    Matthew's Nutrition Service
    Natural Food Mill
    Pasadena's Original Health Food House
POMONA, Nutrition Center

PORTERVILLE, Health Food Center
REDONDO BEACH, Vitamin Bay
REDWOOD CITY, Health Food Center
    Stone's Health Food Center
RENO, Washoe Drug & Health
RESEDA, Reseda Health Foods
RICHMOND, Sayer's
RIVERSIDE, Magnolia Health Center
    Oppliger's
SACRAMENTO, Dane's Public Market
    Elliott's Health Foods
    Health Food Center
    Healthway Specialty Food
    House of Nutrition
    King Karrott Juice Bar
    McAnaw's
    Sacramento Health Foods
SALINAS, Salinas Nutri-Center
SAN BERNARDINO, Harris Co.
    Mac's Health Food Store
SAN CARLOS, San Carlos Health Foods
SAN DIEGO, American Drug Store
    Hillcrest Dietary Foods
    House of Nutrition
    North Park Health Foods
    Physical Therapy
    Plantation Trader's House
    Verd-ee Products
    Vitality Health Food
SAN FERNANDO, Tirrell's
SAN FRANCISCO, Arko Health Food Shop
    Drezdon's Health Foods
    Eat Rite
    G & H Health Foods
    Gala's Health Foods
    Glee's
    Gianette Natural Foods
    Golden Crescent
    Howard's Natural Foods
    Jean's Health Foods
    John's and Jean's

H. L. Johnson Health Foods
King's Health Foods
L. Leonard
McNally's Health Foods
Marina Healthway
Mission Health Foods
National Health Federation
Natural Food Center
Ruth's
Sacramento Health Foods
San Francisco Health Food Store
Sunset Vita Foods
Taraval Health Foods
Vitality Health Foods
SAN JOSE, D & R Dietary Foods
Hale's
Heide's Natural Food Center
Living Foods For Health
Top Notch Nutri-Center
SAN LEANDRO, Hal Stewart's, Health Unlimited
SAN LUIS OBISPO, MacKay's
Margo and Larry's Health Foods
SAN MATEO, Gourmet Healthway
Heide's Healthway
SAN PEDRO, Point Fermin Health Food
SAN RAFAEL, Marin Health Foods
SANTA ANA, Continental Health Foods
Joselle's Health Food Center
SANTA BARBARA, Kayser's
House of Nutrition
Sexauer's
SANTA CRUZ, Health & Diet Foods
Polly Prim Natural Foods
SANTA MONICA, Dietary Foods
Turner's Natural Foods
Vitamin Store
SANTA ROSA, Santa Rosa Health Food Store
SEPULVEDA, Farmer George Market
SHERMAN OAKS, The Health Hut
Logar's Health Foods
Maxon's Drug Co.

Sherman Oaks Nutritional Center
Ventura Medical Pharmacy
SOUTH GATE, Baxter's Health Foods
SOUTH PASADENA, Shattuck's Natural Foods
STOCKTON, Corkery's Nutrition Center
Dane's
Helen's Foods for Health
SUNLAND, Russel James
SUNNYVALE, Healthway Foods
TARZANA, Tarzana Nutritional
TEMPLE CITY, John P. Scherer
Vitality Health Foods
TORRANCE, House of Health
Torrance Health Foods
TUJANGA, Georgi House of Health
TURLOCK, Turlock Health Food Center
TWENTY NINE PALMS, Signe Ohlson Health Foods
VALLEJO, Bell's Foods For Health
VAN NUYS, Van Nuys Health Food Store
VENTURA, Kayser's
VISTA, Erickson Health Foods
Vista Health Foods Store
Wray's
WALNUT CREEK, Kenville Health Foods
WALNUT PARK, Huntington Park Health Foods
WATSONVILLE, Polly Prim Natural Foods
WEST COVINA, House of Health Foods
WEST HOLLYWOOD, Cooley Health Foods
WEST PALM BEACH, Dietetic Vitamin Corp.
WESTWOOD, Westwood Natural Foods
WHITTIER, Whittier Nutrition Center
WILMINGTON, Wilmington Health Foods
WOODLAND, Woodland Nutrition Center
WOODLAND HILLS, West Valley Nutritional Center
YUCAIPA, Shelley's Health Food Store

COLORADO

BOULDER, National Health Food
COLORADO SPRINGS, Specialty Food Shoppe
DENVER, Ethel Barnes Health Food
The Bee Healthy Co.

Denver Health Center
Nidess' Health Food
Vitality Center
ENGLEWOOD, Scientfoods
GRAND JUNCTION, Health Food Center
LAKEWOOD, Lakewood Health Food Store
PUEBLO, Natural Food Center

CONNECTICUT

BRIDGEPORT, Van Dyke's
BRISTOL, Bristol Health Foods
MERIDEN, Meriden Health Center
RIDGEFIELD, Foods
WATERBURY, George T. Dillon
WEST HARTFORD, Alexander's Foods

DISTRICT OF COLUMBIA

WASHINGTON, College Store
J. C. Dimmock
Good Diet Shop
Modern Natural Foods
Olivia's Health Food Service
The Vita Food Company
Woodward & Lothrop

DELAWARE

WILMINGTON, Natural Food Center

FLORIDA

BRADENTON, Dr. Jenkins Health Foods
CLEARWATER, Natural Health Foods
CORAL GABLES, Gables Health Mart
DAYTONA BEACH, Chamberlin Natural Foods
DELAND, Illene's Health Foods
FLORIDA CITY, Suniland Apiaries
FT. LAUDERDALE, Lauderdale Health Food Shop
Gateway Natural Foods
FORT MEYERS, Health Food Mart
Marie's Massage Studio
HOLLYWOOD, Betty's Health Foods

HOMESTEAD, McConnell's Dietetic Foods
    Alfreda's Health Foods
JACKSONVILLE, Diet Shoppe
    Health Food Shop
    Health Food & Vitamin Store
    Natural Vitamin Center
LAKELAND, Natural Food Center
LAKE WORTH, Eve's Natural Foods
MELBOURNE, Emond T. Blazewicz
MIAMI, Bayridge Food Store
    Roy Elkins Health Foods
    Garrett's Health Foods
    Gerrard's Natural Foods
    Mr. Russ Gray
    Miami Vitamin Center
    Murray Health Food Store
    Organic Food Store
    Radiant Health Foods
    Sallye's Natural Foods
    Vitamin Center
MIAMI BEACH, Angelina, Inc.
    Surfside Health Shop
NEW SMYRNA BEACH, Brenzal Groves
ORLANDO, Chamberlin Natural Foods
    Foods For Life of Florida
    Vicompo Corporation
RIVIERA BEACH, Riviera Health Mart
ST. PETERSBURG, Food For Health
    Lewis Health Foods
    Page Foundation
    Vital Food Shop
SARASOTA, Risser's Health Food Shop
    Washburn's Vital Food Shop
TAMPA, Keepwell Nutrition Center
    Bertha Layton's Health Foods
    Tampa Health Food Store
    Tampa Health Food Shop
WEST PALM BEACH, Jack's Health Center
    The Health Food Store
    Jack's Juice Bar

GEORGIA

ATLANTA, Health Food Center
    Health Food Shoppe
    Rosendahl's
    Vital Life Food Center
AUGUSTA, Health Food Store
    H. J. Markwalter's Sons

HAWAII

HONOLULU, Aloha Health Foods
    Chings's Health Foods
    Evans Foods

IDAHO

BOISE, Chase's Health Foods
    Healthway Food Center
BURLEY, Burley Health Food Store
IDAHO FALLS, Thiede Natural Foods
LEWISTON, Lewiston Health Foods
PARMA, Y. Min & Co.
RUPERT, Health Food Center #1
TWIN FALLS, The Sta Well

ILLINOIS

BELLEVILLE, Irma's Kitchen
BENTON, Benton Natural Foods
CHAMPAIGN, Dietary Food Store
CHICAGO, Body Builders Sport Shop
    Braden's
    Chicago Health Food
    Dahl Health Foods
    Eaton's Health Foods Inc.
    Food Consultants
    Dr. Rosalie A. Gusmano
    Health Aids by Page
    Heinrickson's Nee Dee Laboratories
    Hillman's
    Irving Park Health Food
    Henry Junge
    Victor Kaufman Diet Products

Kirn Health Products
Kramer's Health Foods
Logan Diet Foods
Dr. Michael's Health Foods
Montrose Dietary
Morton's Vital Foods, Inc.
National Enzyme Co.
National Health Foods
National Food Center
Nature Food Products
Nichol's Health Foods
Northwest Health Food Center
Nu-Era Health Foods
Pioneer Natural Health Center
Southtown Health Foods
Elizabeth Theiss
Zerrie's System of Health
CICERO, National Health Service
ELGIN, Gromer's Super Markets
EVANSTON, Diet House
Natural & Dietary Foods
HARVEL, A & W Products
MATTOON, Dale von Beheren's Mart
Health Food Shop
Health Food Store
MOLINE, Holdrighe Store
Vitality Foods
NORTHFIELD, Ann's Diet Shelf
OTTAWA, Mel's Market
PEORIA, Peoria Health Food Center
ROCKFORD, Netta Gene Health Foods
Unite Delicatessen
SPRINGFIELD, Jos. T. De Frates Co.
WHEATON, A. G. Dobbins
WILMETTE, W. H. Leahy

INDIANA

ELKHART, W. W. Wilt Co., Inc.
FORT WAYNE, A & B Natural Foods
Geray's
Dr. Lilly Lewellen

GARY, Gary Dietary Foods
    Gary Health Food Center
    Spangle's
HOWE, Pigeon River Gardens
INDIANAPOLIS, Baird Health Products
    Beeler's Natural Foods
    G. & W. Brown Health Foods
    Harry's Natural Food
    Pam's
LAFAYETTE, May's Natural Foods
MICHIGAN CITY, Wilke Drug
SHIPSHEWANA, "Wanna Cup"
TERRE HAUTE, Bon Ton Food Shoppe
WASHINGTON, Barker's Natural Vitamins

IOWA

CEDAR RAPIDS, Jos Barnett & Co.
    Cedar Rapids Health Center
    McCready's Health Foods
    Matteson Health Food Products
DAVENPORT, Federal Health Foods
DES MOINES, Campbell's Foods
    Diet-Wise Health Foods
    Bob's Food Market

KANSAS

COFFEYVILLE, Dillenberger's Natural Food Center
PITTSBURGH, Howard H. Ozburn
SALINAS, Nyles Health Foods
WICHITA, A. B. Health Food Store
    Aunt Anna's Stone Mill—Baker & Natural Foods
    Wichita Health Food Center

KENTUCKY

GLASGOW, Addie's Health Food Shop
LOUISVILLE, Grimm's Diabetic & Diet Foods
    Millen Drug Store
NORTONVILLE, E. F. Oates
OWENSBORO, Robertson's Natural Food Store

LOUISIANA
BATON ROUGE, Health Food Center
  Ogden Park Drugs

MARYLAND
BALTIMORE, Special Diet Shop
TAKOMA PARK, Better Foods Club
  Washington College Store

MASSACHUSETTS
BOSTON, Copley Square Diet Shop
BROOKLINE, Modern Health Shop
CAMBRIDGE, Nature's Food Centers, Inc.
FALL RIVER, The Health Shoppe
GREENFIELD, Miss Dee Archambault
MELROSE, Melrose Health Food
NEW BEDFORD, Seaplant Foods
PLYMOUTH, Natural Food Shop
QUINCY, Health Food Center
SALEM, Health Food Store
SOMERSET, The Health Shoppe
SOMERVILLE, Healthway Food Shoppe
SPRINGFIELD, Goyette Health Food and Specialty Shoppe
WOLLASTON, Modern Foods Inc.

MICHIGAN
DEARBORN, Health Food Center
BAY CITY, Emily's Health Foods
DETROIT, Detroit Vital Foods
    Lloyd H. Elrod
    Harwith Health Foods
    Health Champions
    Health Supreme Foods
    J. L. Hudson Co.
    Mac's Health Foods
    Martin's Health Foods
    Moore's Health Foods
    Nature's Way
    Nutrition Brands
    Jos. Pocock & Sons

Rim Nutrition Brands
St. Jean Beaupre Health
Sawall Health Foods
Sawall Natural Products
Shedd-Bartusch Foods
Elizabeth Sewall Strahan
Vita Health Shop
Vita Nook Health Foods
Wonder Foods
EAST TOWES, Cosadd's Manna Shop
EVERETT, Everett Health Foods
FLINT, Dale's Natural Foods
    Del's Foods
FORT HURON, Detroit Tea Store
GRAND RAPIDS, Nature's Health Foods
    Gordon F. Sawall Health Foods
    Sawall Natural Health Foods
    Stone Mill Products Co.
HIGHLAND PARK, Marlin Health Food Shop
HIGHLANDS, Voegeles Health Foods
JACKSON, Henry's Pure Food Shop
KALAMAZOO, Town & Country Super Market
LANSING, Gibbs Natural Foods
    Randall's Health Foods
    Sawall Health Foods Products
LIVONIA, Zerbo's Health Foods
MOUNT CLEMENS, Health Food Store
MUNSING, Ann's Health Shop
PONTIAC, Natural Health Foods
RICHMOND, Ridge Health Foods
ROYAL OAK, Nutri Foods
    Royal Oak Nutrition
SAGINAW, Home Dairy Co.
TRAVERSE CITY, Food Specialties Shop
VICKSBURG, Jericho Foods

MINNESOTA

MINNEAPOLIS, Cayol Foods Center
    Frances Freeman
    Organic Products Inc.

The Paro Co.
Pavo's Foods

MISSISSIPPI

GULFPORT, Garon's Fine Foods
PHILADELPHIA, Mrs. Chisholm's Candies

MISSOURI

INDEPENDENCE, Staff O'Life Health Foods
JOPLIN, C. R. Hunt
KANSAS CITY, Chatman's Special Foods
    Coffey's Health Foods
    National Vitamin & Mineral Store
    Natural Food Center
    The Pantry Shelf
NEOSHO, Natural Food Store
NEVADA, Nevada Health Foods
ST. JOSEPH, Holsum Health Food Store
ST. LOUIS, New Dawn Vital Foods
    Organic Food Service
    Geo. C. Tong Co.
    The Vitamin Store
SPRINGFIELD, Evans Health Studio
    Health Food Store
    Vital Foods Service

MONTANA

BILLINGS, Schroeder's Health Center
GREAT FALLS, Fountain Of Youth Health Foods

NEBRASKA

LINCOLN, Health Food Service
    Lincoln Health Food Center
OMAHA, Health Food Service
    Thomas Kilpatrick

NEVADA

LAS VEGAS, Siemen's Health Foods
RENO, Jackwill's Natural Foods
SPARKS, Guerian Sales
    Wehaveit Shop

NEW JERSEY

ASBURY PARK, Hill's Drug Store
ATLANTIC CITY, Jay Brown Natural Foods
BEACHWOOD, Nature's Way To Health
BERGENFIELD, The Health Shoppe
CAMDEN, Ostrov's Food Center
EAST ORANGE, Olive May Co.
  Wayne Coffee Co.
ELIZABETH, All Diet Health Foods
  Diet Shop
  The Diet Shop Inc.
HACKENSACK, Aylward's Health Center
HADDON HEIGHTS, Low's Foods
IRVINGTON, Irvington Health Food Center
JERSEY CITY, Advanced Health Foods
  Jaxon Health Foods
  Lordell Health Foods
  Natur Rite
KEARNY, Kearny Health Foods
MORRISTOWN, The Health Shoppe
NEWARK, A B C Health Foods
  Zinn's Health Foods
PASSAIC, Dietary Food Service
  Dietary Health Foods
  Dobrin's Pharmacy
PATERSON, Felicia's Vital Food Service
  Vital Food Service
PLAINFIELD, Plainfield Health Food Service
RED BANK, Perry's Natural Foods
SUMMIT, Summit Health Food Center
TRENTON, Special Foods Centre

NEW MEXICO

ALBUQUERQUE, Fountain Of Health
  Radiant Health Products
  Shop For Better Health
SANTA FE, Aztec Studio
  The Health Food Shop
TRUTH OR CONSEQUENCES, Health Food Store

NEW YORK

ALBANY, Nature Food Center
    Van Dyke
AMSTERDAM, Stanley Dietetic Foods
AUBURN, Gus Nestopoulos
BAYSIDE, Bayside Health & Specialty Foods
BINGHAMTON, Gift-Gourmet-Shop
BUFFALO, Hauser Health Foods
    Healthful Diet Shoppe
    Margaret's Health Food Shoppe
    O'Toole's Dietary Foods
ELMIRA, Iza Ostrander Foods
HEMPSTEAD, Pullman Diet Foods
    Pullman Diet Shop
HUNTINGTON, Huntington Diet Foods
MAMARONECK, Mamaroneck Diet & Health
MOUNT VERNON, Lo-Cal Diet Shop
NEW ROCHELLE, Natural Health Foods
NEW YORK CITY: Bronx, Anshen & Gertler
    Bronx Coffee Co.
    Fordham Health Foods
    H. & R. Health Foods
    Martin Health Shop
    Mello's Health Foods
    Merton Health Foods
    Mollo's Natural Food Shoppe
  Brooklyn: Approved Organic Foods
    Harry's Health Food Stores
    Live 'n Health
    Mitty's Health Foods
    Pearls of Health Foods
    Skandia Health Food Store
    David Solomon
    Stamina Health Foods
    Sturdee Food Products
    Traymore Food Shop
    Vigor, Inc.
  Manhattan: A-1 Health Foods
    A-Radiant Health Foods
    Acadia Natural Foods

All Diet Foods
All Health Foods Distributors
Baum Health Service
Better Diet Shop
Brownies Natural Food Products
Damers Natural Foods
B. Fannekchl
Health Foods
Health Haven
Healthway Shops
Honey House
Kubie's Health Foods
Lake States Yeast Food
Lust's Health Foods
Mary Lust's Health Food Shop
New Health Foods
Organic Health Foods, Inc.
Organic Natural Foods
Riedel Food Products Co.
Salad Bowl
Sunny Health Foods
Vitality Health Foods
Vitamin Bar
Vim & Vigor
Yorkville Health Foods
Queens: Flushing, Sunrise Health Foods
Long Island City, Astoria Health Food Center
STATEN ISLAND, Walter L. White
Staten Island Health Food
NIAGARA FALLS, Niagara Health Food Center
POUGHKEEPSIE, Poughkeepsie Food Center
ROCHESTER, Dietary Specialties
Fountain Of Youth
Healthful Diet Shoppe
Nature Food Centres
SCHENECTADY, Patton's Health Foods
SPRING VALLEY, Hilda Van's Health Foods
SYRACUSE, American Health Center
Healthful Diet Shop
Vegetable Products Co.

TROY, Troy Nutritious Foods, Inc.
VESTAL, Arnold's Health Products

NORTH CAROLINA

ASHEVILLE, The Good Health Place
CHARLOTTE, Elliot's Health Foods

NORTH DAKOTA

FARGO, Leeby's Food Market

OHIO

AKRON, Alexander Health Foods
ALLIANCE, Market Grocery
BEDFORD, Margie's Juice Bar & Restaurant
CANTON, Royer Health Foods
    Schauer's Health Food Center
CINCINNATI, Parks-Phillipps Foods
    Spatz Health Foods
CLEVELAND, Chandler & Rudd
    Hobart Health Foods
    The House of Health
    Vitality Health Food Shop
    Vita-Mart
COLUMBUS, Haigis Health Foods
    Weigand Health Foods
CUYAHOGA FALLS, State Rd. Health Food Center
DAYTON, Dayton Natural Foods
    Hannah Early
    Irene's Health Food Shop
LAKEWOOD, Marshall Health Foods
MANSFIELD, Variety Outlet
NEW PHILADELPHIA, Klar Health Foods
NORTH CANTON, Noebe's Health Food Shoppe
OLMSTEAD FALLS, Natural Foods Inc.
    Natural Food Institute
SANDUSKY, Fireland Grist Mill
SPRINGFIELD, Williams' House Of Foods
TIFFIN, Tiffin Health Food Store
TOLEDO, Dietrich's Health Foods
    Eisenmann's Health Foods

WARREN, Ideal Health Foods
YOUNGSTOWN, Health Food Center
Natural Health Foods

OKLAHOMA

CLAREMORE, Dickerson Health Foods
OKLAHOMA CITY, The Diet Shop
Nutritional Food Center
Tauscher's Natural Foods
TULSA, Akins Health Foods
Earl's Health Center

OREGON

ALBANY, Albany Natural Food Shop
ASHLAND, Pine Knoll Natural Products
Twin Oaks Foods
COOS BAY, Coos Bay Health Food Store
EUGENE, Nutrition Center
GLADSTONE, Staff O'Life Foods
GRANT'S PASS, Massie's Natural Foods
KLAMATH FALLS, Holden's
MEDFORD, Nutrition Foods Center
Rouge Valley Natural Foods
OSWEGO, Specialty Food Shop
PORTLAND, Bio Chemic Foods
Boyse Grocery Health Store
Brammert's Radiant Health Food
Healthway Food Center
Nutrition Food Center
Ross Vital Foods
ROSEBURG, Roseburg Natural Foods
Umpqua Health Foods
SALEM, J. L. Busick & Son
Welth's Health Center
SPRINGFIELD, Ferguson's Health Foods

PENNSYLVANIA

ALLENTOWN, Natural Foods Specialty Center
C. E. Shaffer Specialty Foods
ARDMORE, Main Line Diet Shop

AUBURN, Diebert & Young
 Natural Health Food Store
BEAVER FALLS, Nu Age Health Center
BETHLEHEM, Parker's Grocery Company
DENVER, Weaver's Health Foods
EAST PITTSBURGH, Dr. Frank Abbate, M.D.
ERIE, Dietetic Food Company
 Hilda Kuhn's Health Food Store
FEASTERVILLE, Alladan Farms
HANOVER, Health Foods
HARRISBURG, De-Lite Health Store
 Golden Rule Food Shop
 LeFevre Health Food Center
JOHNSTOWN, Poulsen's
LANCASTER, Natural Food Store
 Wenger's
McMURRAY, Nu-Age Biogranic Products
PALMYRA, Dietary & Natural Foods
 Palmyra Health Store
PENNSBURG, Sproutmatic Research
PENNS CREEK, Walnut Acres
PHILADELPHIA, Better Diet Shop
 Gimbel Bros.
 Lahr's Nutri-Food Center
 Low's Food Store
 Thomas Martindale Co.
 Nature Food Centers
 Olney Health Food Co.
PITTSBURGH, Dewalt Health Foods
 East Liberty Health Food Shop
 Lackzoon Health Foods
 Lackzoon Health Stores
POTTSTOWN, Kay's Shop
READING, Home of Natural Foods
 R. F. Natural Foods
SWARTHMORE, The Nut House
SCHOENECK, Mease's Natural Foods
SCRANTON, Natural Food Center
VENETIA, Ceriatrex Products Co.
WIRETON, Hainley's Special Diet Foods
YORK, Apollo Health Store

RHODE ISLAND

PAWTUCKET, Adam's Drug Company

SOUTH DAKOTA

HURON, Health Food Shop

TENNESSEE

COLLEGEDALE, College Enterprises
KNOXVILLE, Natural Foods
MEMPHIS, Health Food Store
    Healthway Food Store

TEXAS

ABILENE, Morris-Daniels
AMARILLO, Eat Rite Health Foods
ARLINGTON, Realife Foods
AUSTIN, Austin Natural Foods
    The Health Kitchen
    Nutrilite Foods
BEAUMONT, Adams Dietary Foods
BORGER, Worley Health Foods
BROWNWOOD, Brownwood Dietetic Store
BRYANT, The Pantry
CORPUS CHRISTI, Jane's Health Foods
DALLAS, Clark's Health Foods
    Dallas Health Food Center
    Plaza Health Foods Store
EL PASO, McKee Prescription
    Vitamin Store
FT. WORTH, Health & Realife Diet Foods
    Lifanu
    Monnigs Health Foods
GREGGTON, Natural Food Center
HARLINGTON, Harlington Health Foods
HOUSTON, American Health Food Co.
    Dixie Health Food Cottage
    Highland Village Health Foods
    Natural Food Center
    Sunshine Health Foods
    Vitamin Specialties Co.
IRVING, Lazy A. Ranch

LUBBOCK, Blackburn Health Foods
    Grace Health Foods
PECOS, Cline's Health Foods
PORT ARTHUR, Plettman's
SAN ANGELO, Schantz Health Foods
SAN ANTONIO, Certified Health Foods
    Harmon's Health Food Service
    Moore Natural Food Works
    Sterling Natural Foods
TEXARKANA, Natural Health Foods
TYLER, Avis Health Foods
WACO, Health Food Store
WICHITA FALLS, Diet Food Shoppe

UTAH

BOUNTIFUL, Clinton's Wheat Shop
OGDEN, Goddart's Health Mart
PROVO, College Health Food Store
SALT LAKE CITY, J. W. Broadwater
    Clinton's Sta Well
    Henry's Juice Co.
    Irene's Natural Health Food Store
    People's Health Foods
    Scheibner Health Foods
    Sta-Well Health Store
    Sta-Well Natural Foods
    Z.C.M.I.

VIRGINIA

ALEXANDRIA, Health Food Center
COPPER HILL, Copper Hill Sales Service
DAYTON, Nutritional Foods, Inc.
    Thomas Home Bakery
RICHMOND, Richmond Health Food Center

WASHINGTON

BELLINGHAM, Bellingham Health House
    Vitality Food Center
BREMERTON, Healthways
    Helen's Natural Foods
    Healthways

CHEHALIS, Roundtree H. Center
EVERETT, Everett Health Foods
KENNEWICK, Tri-City Natural Foods
MOUNT VERNON, Dolan Vital Foods
    Thompson's Vital Foods
OLYMPIA, Gifford's Country Store
    Sta-Well Health Service
OPPORTUNITY, Cottage Shop
PUYALLUP, Luckows Health Service
SEATTLE, Brewster's Health Service
    Burien Special Foods
    Cook's Finer Foods
    Cook's Natural Foods
    Jerome's Natural Foods
    Lenora's Natural Foods
    Dr. McCormick's Natl. Foods
    Pioneer Natural Foods
    Security Health Foods
    Western Natural Foods Co.
SPOKANE, Hoss Modern Foods
    Raymond Natural Foods
    Spokane Nutrition Center
TACOMA, Conklin's Nutritional
    Groff's Natural Foods
    Saunders Health Service
    Treasure House
YAKIMA, Beem's Diet Food Center
    Yakima Natural Foods
VANCOUVER, Vancouver Health Food Center

WEST VIRGINIA

FAIRMONT, A & M Dietetic Foods

WISCONSIN

APPLETON, Steger Nutrition Centre
BELOIT, Krezin's Garden Shop
GREEN BAY, Leroy Health Center
    Mollenhauer Vitamins, Inc.
KENOSHA, Kenosha Natural Foods
    Kenosha Nutritional Foods
MADISON, Vital Foods Inc.

MANITOWOC, Health Food Shop
  Neff's Health Food Shop
MEDFORD, Medford Health Foods
MILWAUKEE, Bergholz House of Health
  Ceil's Specialty Foods
  Colonial Health Foods
  Family Health Store
  Katherine's Dietetic Shop
  Kitchen Craft-Dietary Shop
  Langlois Health Food Mart
  Natural Food Shop
  Natural Foods
SHEBOYGAN, Frank Pungarcher
  Steger Nutritional Foods

WYOMING

SHERIDAN, Kirkpatrick Health